D1741035

Mild Hypertension: is there pressure to treat?

An account of the MRC trial
by W. E. Miall and Gillian Greenberg
on behalf of
The Medical Research Council's
Working Party on
Mild to Moderate Hypertension

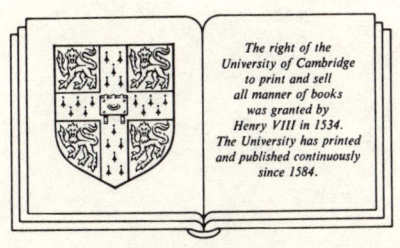

The right of the
University of Cambridge
to print and sell
all manner of books
was granted by
Henry VIII in 1534.
The University has printed
and published continuously
since 1584.

CAMBRIDGE UNIVERSITY PRESS
Cambridge
London   New York   New Rochelle
Melbourne   Sydney

Published by the Press Syndicate of the University of Cambridge
The Pitt Building, Trumpington Street, Cambridge CB2 1RP
32 East 57th Street, New York, NY 10022, USA
10 Stamford Road, Oakleigh, Melbourne 3166, Australia

© Cambridge University Press 1987

First published 1987

Printed in Great Britain at
the University Press, Cambridge

British Library cataloguing in publication data

Miall, W. E.
Mild hypertension: is there pressure to treat? An account of the
MRC trial.
1. Hypertension
I. Title   II. Greenberg, Gillian
III. Medical Research Council (*Working
Party on Mild to Moderate Hypertension)*
616.1'32   RC685.H8

Library of Congress cataloging in publication data

Miall, W. E.
Mild hypertension: is there pressure to treat?
Bibliography
1. Hypertension – Chemotherapy – Evaluation.
2. Hypotensive agents – Testing.   I. Greenberg, Gillian.
II. Medical Research Council (Great Britain). Working
Party on Mild to Moderate Hypertension.   III. Title.
[DNLM: 1. Clinical Trials. 2. Hypertension – drug
therapy. WG 340 M6175m]
RC685.H8M5   1986   616.1'32061   86-18842

ISBN 0 521 33293 1

Contents

Foreword

There can be few principles that are more generally approved and more consistently ignored than the principle that prevention is better than cure. Given the choice between suffering from a disease and being cured or avoiding the disease altogether only a masochist would, other things being equal, choose the former. Other things, however, seldom are equal and individuals and societies frequently prefer to accept risks, even when the resulting diseases do not respond to treatment, than to take the steps that are needed to avoid them.

This, of course, is not surprising, as the activities that cause disease may be pleasant, useful, or economically rewarding, while those needed for its prevention are sometimes unpleasant, costly, or productive of other risks of a possibly more immediate sort. Sometimes too the risks may be felt to be very different from what they actually are and the balance of advantage and disadvantage is commonly determined less by objective assessment than by subjective perception. Often, however, the extent of the real risks can be only guessed at, judgments may vary, and hazards that might be easily avoided continue to cause premature death and unnecessary suffering.

This certainly seemed to be the case with regard to the detection and treatment of moderately raised blood pressure, of the order of 140 to 180 mm Hg systolic or 90 to 109 mm Hg diastolic, when, in 1970, a group of clinicians asked the Medical Research Council to fund a trial to find out precisely what the benefits and costs might be, if all people with pressures at this level could be identified and treated on a national scale. It was not, however, any easy problem to tackle. For the events that clinicians were seeking to learn how to avoid occur infrequently and are important to avoid only because their effect is so devastating if they do unfortunately occur. Many thousands of participants were, therefore, needed, each of whom had to be sufficiently enthused by the object of the study to follow a strict regime and to remain under observation for many years without even knowing whether the medicine that was prescribed contained any active ingredient.

It speaks, therefore, very highly of the Council's concern for the practical application of research results that the study was funded for so long, despite the continued drain on its resources, and very highly of the efficiency of the organisers and of their ability to communicate that it was initiated and carried through to a successful conclusion. But to those of us who are concerned with preventive medicine and would like to see greater efforts put into the prevention of disease, not because it will save money but because it is something to be desired in itself, the successful conclusion of the study speaks even more highly of the opportunities for the future. For it tells us that thousands of people are sufficiently interested in health and concerned for the public good to collaborate with general practitioners and nurses in a serious attempt to discover how to prevent disease, even at the cost of considerable personal inconvenience and trouble. And it tells us, too, that it is possible to obtain useful quantitative information about the effect of a method of prevention that would be of value on a national scale, even if it produces only a moderate reduction in the extent of the risk to an individual.

1986   Richard Doll

Preface

Writing a book on behalf of a committee is less traumatic than might be imagined. Perhaps we were just fortunate. Our colleagues had valuable ideas and suggestions, and were helpful in redrafting the more obscure parts of our text.

The book is a record of what came to be known as 'the' MRC trial. The Medical Research Council has, of course, conducted many other therapeutic trials; some of them have produced more clear-cut answers to the questions being asked than did this one. Nonetheless, it was an important trial and it generated a lot of interest. This was largely because mild hypertension is an international problem of concern to 5 or 10% of the adult population; it is a condition which underlies much of the twentieth century's epidemic of cardiovascular disease.

We delayed the publication of this book until the major papers giving the trial's results had appeared in the journals; but there may be dozens of useful papers which could and should be written on different aspects of the results and to await the last of them would delay this volume until it had lost all topical interest.

The book is likely to be of value to a rather specialised readership. Those involved with large-scale randomised trials may find the descriptions of the organisation of this study of interest and they will not find the details of the logistics elsewhere. They may also welcome hearing about the ethical problems we encountered. Future trials for mild hypertension will pose new questions and the ethical issues may make the conduct of them more difficult as evidence accumulates that treatment does confer certain benefits.

Physicians and others concerned with hypertension may appreciate the opportunity to examine the findings in one volume without needing to peruse copies of several different journals. But the book is not the sort which a medical student faced with finals in three months time should be advised to study.

Readers will certainly find results here which are difficult to interpret; that is perhaps a good reason for including them. Even within the MRC Working Party, and between the two authors, there were differences of interpretation of the results and different views on what should and what should not be written about them. Some of the findings were not part of the original design, were unexpected and will need confirmation. They are none the less interesting for that.

May 1986   W. E. M. and G. G.

Acknowledgments

A great many people contributed to this study in a wide variety of ways. We thank them all and apologise to those whose names should be, but are not, listed below; the largest group are the 17 354 patients who helped by their participation in the trial.

Others closely involved with different aspects of the work included Patrick Brennan who, with some help from Simon Thompson, was responsible for all the computing and statistical control; Tom Whitehead and his colleagues at the Wolfson Research Laboratories who undertook the biochemical work; Hugh Tunstall Pedoe who assessed events; Anthony Mann and Paul Whelton who supervised the psychiatric and 24-hour ECG monitoring studies, respectively; Jean Wilderspin, Jill Fisher and their team at the co-ordinating centre; Greta Barnes and Wendy Browne who at different times led the team of training nurses – Pam Allen, Jean Barton, Sue Drummond, Margaret Goldsborough, Daphne Hammond, Leslie Hand, Elaine Kacser, Margaret McGowan, Eileen Marshall, Audrey Miller, Kay Penny and the late Penny Mitchell; and Joy Cater. Richard Bowlby and the Department of Medical Illustration at Northwick Park, with computing from Lawrence Miall, provided almost all the artwork.

Thanks are also due to the four pharmaceutical companies who provided drugs and a great deal of financial support – Imperial Chemical Industries Ltd, Glaxo Operations U.K. Ltd, Ciba Laboratories and Merck Sharp and Dohme Ltd.

Pauline Howlett, with characteristic patience and good humour, was responsible for preparing the text for publication. We are indeed grateful for the help of so many kind friends.

The MRC Working Party

Members of the Working Party
Professor Sir Stanley Peart (chairman), Mrs G. R. Barnes (until 1983), Mr P. M. G. Broughton, Professor A. L. Cochrane (until 1977), Professor C. T. Dollery, Dr K. G. Green (until 1983), Dr J.

F. Harrison (until 1977), Professor W. W. Holland (until 1977), Dr
M. F. Hudson, Dr D. M. Humphreys (until 1978), Dr A. F. Lever,
Dr T. W. Meade, Dr W. E. Miall (secretary until 1983), Professor G.
A. Rose, the late Dr B. C. Smith (until 1980), Dr P. Wilding (until
1977), and Dr G. Greenberg (secretary).

Members of the Monitoring Committee
Professor G. A. Rose (chairman), Dr M. W. Adler (until 1978), Mr
P. J. Brennan, Dr E. C. Coles (until 1978), Dr G. Greenberg, Dr M.
Hamilton, Dr J. A. Heady, Dr T. W. Meade, Dr W. E. Miall, Dr
E. B. Raftery (until 1978), Mr S. G. Thompson (until 1984),
Professor H. D. Tunstall Pedoe.

Members of the Ethical Committee
Professor Sir Richard Doll (chairman), Dr J. Fry, Dr M. Hamilton
(until 1980), Dr J. A. Heady (until 1980), Professor Sir Raymond
Hoffenberg, Professor J. H. Ledingham, Dr P. J. Taylor.

Co-ordinating Centre Staff
Dr W. E. Miall, Dr G. Greenberg, Mr P. J. Brennan, Mr S. G.
Thompson, Dr T. W. Meade, Mrs C. W. Browne, Mrs J. Wilderspin,
Mrs J. Fisher, Mrs S. Collins, Mrs P. Denness, Mrs A. Duquesne,
Mrs V. Egan, Mrs J. Farnham, Mrs O. Fuller, Mrs M. Hamnett, Mrs
P. Jenkins, Mrs M. McCann, Mrs M. Morris, Miss M. Richards,
Miss S. Sinha, Mrs Y. Speight, the late Miss S. Standring.

ECG Readers
Mrs C. Rose, Mrs N. Keen, Dr G. Greenberg, Dr W. E. Miall, Dr
M. Farooqi, Mrs D. Marston, L. S. Miall, Miss J. Tudhope, Dr J. D.
Williams.

General Practices
Abingdon, Oxfordshire. Dr R. S. Pinches, Mrs J. Barton, Mrs W.
    Dolling.
Abingdon, Oxfordshire. Dr J. W. K. Ward, Mrs W. Dolling.
Aintree, Merseyside. Dr J. M. Forrest, Mrs M. Murphy.
Alconbury, Huntingdonshire. Dr P. Sackin, Mrs J. Rogers, Mrs A.
    Allen.
Aldeburgh, Suffolk. Dr I. Tait, Mrs M. Tate.
Alexandria, Dunbartonshire. Dr A. L. Black, Dr A. Baxter, Mrs M.
    McGowan.
Alresford, Hampshire. Dr G. C. Brill, Mrs M. Mackrell, Mrs S.
    Clark.
Ashington, Northumberland. Dr A. Hutchinson, Mrs J. Thompson,
    Mrs H. Elliott.

Backwell, Avon. Dr K. W. Miller, Mrs M. Chivers.

Banstead, Surrey. Dr C. M. Molloy, Dr M. Ahmed, Mrs P. Jones.

Barnsley, Yorkshire. Dr J. D. Williamson, Dr A. O'Carroll, Mrs J. Littlewood.

Barnstaple, Devon. Dr I. M. F. Jack, Dr P. Lippiett, Mrs S. Footner, Mrs M. Cooper.

Barnstaple, Devon. Dr J. G. Turner, Mrs P. Turner.

Barton-on-Humber, Lincolnshire. Dr J. Pemberton, Mrs D. Curtis.

Basildon, Essex. Dr P. B. Martin, Mrs D. Bass.

Bath, Avon. Dr A. A. Graham, Dr G. D. Walker, Mrs M. Goldsborough, Mrs J. Head.

Bath, Avon. Dr R. L. King, Mrs P. Bennett.

Bath, Avon. Dr R. L. Rolls, Mrs M. Holton.

Beaconsfield, Buckinghamshire. Dr D. Gau, Dr S. Cox, Mrs M. Crawford, Mrs V. Marsden.

Bicester, Oxfordshire. Dr R. Macleod, Mrs D. Stephenson.

Bideford, Devon. Dr E. W. M. Channing, Dr M. Cracknell, Mrs M. Cracknell.

Bidford on Avon, Warwickshire. Dr J. Cavanagh, Mrs M. Record.

Bishops Lydeard, Somerset. Dr R. Harrison, Mrs H. Salway.

Blackheath, London. Dr J. Wood, Mrs A. Watson, Mrs S. Knight.

Bletchley, Northamptonshire. Dr B. R. Patel, Miss G. Hallett.

Bournemouth, Hampshire. Dr M. D. Johnson, Mrs J. Masters.

Bracknell, Berkshire. Dr M. W. Robinson, Mrs P. Allen.

Bromsgrove, W. Midlands. Dr A. V. Cowan, Dr R. C. W. Wynne, Mrs E. Woolf.

Bude, Cornwall. Dr D. Giles, Mrs S. Kershaw.

Bungay, Suffolk. Dr C. H. Hand, Mrs L. Hand.

Burton on Trent, Staffordshire. Dr J. Gilberthorpe, Mrs M. Hale, Mrs S. Drummond.

Camberley, Surrey. Dr A. M. W. Porter, Mrs J. Smith.

Cambridge. Dr P. Eckstein, Mrs C. Kaufman, Mrs V. Zarno.

Cambridge. Dr J. B. Hickling, Mrs J. Wilkins.

Cambridge. Dr H. King, Mrs D. Barlow.

Cardiff, Glamorgan. Dr D. A. Cadman, Mrs U. Clark.

Carnforth, Lancashire. Dr J. Shakespeare, Mrs M. Hignett.

Carnoustie, Tayside. Dr H. Leslie, Mrs V. Hunter.

Castle Douglas, Dumfriesshire. Dr I. Carmichael, Dr A. P. D. Wilkinson, Mrs A. Farish.

Catford, London. Dr R. L. Meyrick, Sister M. Bone.

Chertsey, Surrey. Dr G. A. Hobbs, Dr P. F. Brodribb, Mrs J. Kidd.

Chessington, Surrey. Dr M. S. Udal, Mrs B. Seymour.

Chesterfield, Derbyshire. Dr R. A. Mee, Mrs P. Mitchell.

Chislehurst, Kent. Dr R. May, Mrs S. Knight.

Cleckheaton, Yorkshire. Dr G. Worrall, Dr M. S. A. Khan, Mrs J. Lamb.

Cleobury Mortimer, Shropshire. Dr D. Nixon, Mrs G. Cuming.

Clitheroe, Lancashire. The late Dr G. Hampson, Mrs J. Pyatt, Mrs M. Dobson.

Coleford, Somerset. Dr D. Rawlins, Dr D. C. Thomson, Mrs H. Andrews, Mrs M. G. Peers.

Corstorphine, Edinburgh. Dr H. V. Edwards, Mrs A. Wood.

Corstorphine, Edinburgh. Dr D. Holton, Mrs M. Macmillan.

Crawley, Sussex. Dr G. Strube, Mrs L. Holt.

Crowthorne, Berkshire. Dr W. J. H. Lord, Mrs M. Clark.

Dalbeattie, Kirkcudbrightshire. Dr E. Rose, Mrs J. McAdam.

Darley Dale, Derbyshire. Dr C. R. Martys, Mrs B. Greaves.

Denbigh, Clwyd. Dr P. L. Hackett, Mrs E. Thomas.

Dingwall, Highland. Dr A. A. A. McCall, Mrs E. Low.

Dumfries. Dr W. A. M. Wilson, Mrs A. Farish.

Dunstable, Bedfordshire. Dr H. D. Bodhani, Mrs M. Smither, Mrs D. Thompson.

Durham. Dr R. H. C. Catty, Mrs B. Blake.

Eastbourne, Sussex. Dr V. Gurney, Mrs J. Rowlands, Mrs C. A. Pickering.

Edenbridge, Kent. Dr T. R. L. Bailey, Mrs K. Knott, Mrs Y. Elliott.

Englefield Green, Surrey. Dr G. A. E. Baker, Mrs H. Elliott.

Edinburgh. Dr P. G. White, Mrs E. Kacser.

Enfield, Middlesex. Dr A. T. Ridge, Mrs A. Porter.

Evesham, Worcestershire. Dr G. Burton, Mrs E. Wray, Mrs A. Davis.

Exmouth, Devon. Dr D. M. Humphreys, Dr C. A. Stubbings, Miss D. Hammond.

Fareham, Hampshire. Dr K. Barnard, Mrs J. Wilkes.

Farnborough, Hampshire. Dr N. R. Sales, Mrs B. O'Callaghan, Mrs P. White.

Folkestone, Kent. Dr G. T. Whitaker, the late Mrs P. Mitchell, Mrs M. Edey, Mrs M. Moore.

Four Oaks, West Midlands. Dr D. F. J. Archer, Mrs K. Hough, Mrs J. Homer.

Frodsham, Cheshire. Dr G. J. Dickinson, Mrs J. Dickinson.

Gloucester. Dr J. B. Peniket, Mrs S. Arnold, Mrs B. James

Gorseinon, West Glamorgan. Dr D. J. Davies, Dr B. Evans, Mrs H. Upton.

Gosforth, Tyne and Wear. Dr P. A. Dodds, Mrs M. Dodds.

Guisborough, Cleveland. Dr D. C. Marr, Mrs A. Williams.

Halesworth, Suffolk. Dr G. I. Mair, Mrs L. Downing.

Handforth, Cheshire. Dr S. M. Johnson, Mrs W. Lewis, Mrs A. Long.

Harrogate, Yorkshire. Dr J. Heatley, Mrs D. Thomas.

Heacham, Norfolk. Dr I. K. Campbell, Mrs B. Blacklock.

Henley on Thames, Oxfordshire. Dr A. H. Melhuish, Mrs N. Girling.

Herne Bay, Kent. Dr J. N. Brown, Dr R. Wheeldon, Mrs S. Enright.

High Wycombe, Buckinghamshire. Dr J. Horner, Dr D. Scott, Mrs C. Weeks.

Highams Park, London. Dr G. F. Norris, Sister B. Sankey.

Hildenborough, Kent. Dr W. D. Callum, Mrs R. Ford, Mrs M. Romney.

Holmes Chapel, Cheshire. Dr M. F. Hudson, Mrs M. Davies, Mrs P. Farrance.

Horwich, Lancashire. Dr P. J. Ellis, Mrs E. Marshall.

Hoyland, S. Yorkshire. Dr D. J. Fairclough, Mrs R. Walker.

Inverness, Highland. Dr H. I. McNamara, Mrs S. MacIntosh.

Ipswich, Suffolk. Dr D. Meldrum, Miss J. Osborne.

Keadby, Lincolnshire. Dr J. Zacharias, Mrs C. Sinclair.

Keighley, Yorkshire. Dr R. G. Morey, Dr A. P. Harrison, Mrs A. Gunton.

Keynsham, Avon. Dr N. R. Nutt, Mrs J. Mills.

Keynsham, Avon. Dr J. Wyatt, Mrs M. Holton.

Kidderminster, Worcestershire. Dr J. M. Wilner, Mrs E. Ford.

Kidderminster, Worcestershire. Dr V. Schrieber, Mrs J. Watkins.

Kilsyth, Stirlingshire. Dr P. A. Sandham, Mrs Z. G. Fleming, Mrs A. McLanachan.

Leamington Spa, Warwickshire. Dr J. Martyrossian, Mrs J. Furnell, Mrs M. Scott.

Leeds, Yorkshire. Dr J. R. Jeffrey, Mrs J. Bannan, Mrs P. Leatham.

Leiston, Suffolk. Dr K. Osler, Mrs M. Tate.

Lenham, Kent. Dr I. D. H. McMullen, Mrs E. Porter.

Lightwater, Surrey. Dr F. de S. Donnan, Mrs E. Pierssene.

Liverpool. Dr M. Goodman, Mrs D. Darnton, Mrs M. Iball.

Liverpool. Dr C. Taylor, Dr A. M. W. Forbes, Mrs J. Norman.

Livingston, Midlothian. Dr M. P. Ryan, Mrs C. Coupar.

Loughborough, Leicestershire. Dr K. J. Evans, Mrs J. Greer.

Lyminge, Kent. Dr M. P. B. Jones, Mrs J. B. Jones.

Macclesfield, Cheshire. Dr J. D. Broadbent, Sister K. Lowe.

Macclesfield, Cheshire. Dr P. Baker, Dr J. Fletcher, Mrs P. M. Cameron.

Maghull, Merseyside. Dr R. A. Yorke, Mrs R. Denny.

Mansfield, Nottinghamshire. Dr J. J. Hennessy, Mrs M. Sanderson, Mrs R. Thorpe.

Marlborough, Wiltshire. Dr R. A. Reekie, Mrs J. Nightingale, Mrs A. Bew.

Maryport, Cumbria. Dr K. Longstaff, Mrs C. Thompson.

Midsomer Norton, Avon. Dr J. P. Valentine, Dr J. G. Davies, Mrs J. Charlton.

Musselburgh, Midlothian. Dr A. D. Watson, Dr I. Johnston, Mrs Z. Eunson.

Nailsea, Avon. Dr D. P. Wright, Mrs M. Chivers.

Neston, Wirral. Dr J. W. McCrone, Dr M. Perry, Mrs S. Kennedy.

Newbold, Derbyshire. Dr S. C. Gillam, Mrs S. Cresswell.

Newmarket, Cambridgeshire. Dr A. J. S. White, Mrs F. Morris.

Northampton. Dr T. J. Gill, Mrs A. Broadhurst.

Northampton. Dr D. Gillam, Dr J. Fenton, Mrs H. Fenton.

Nuneaton, West Midlands. Dr K. L. H. Flynn, Mrs J. Joyce, Mrs F. Howell, Mrs L. Waite, Mrs N. Harrop.

Ongar, Essex. Dr B. Rix, Mrs P. Nicol.

Oxford. Dr R. Lloyd, Mrs R. Milnes.

Pencoed, West Glamorgan. Dr W. Phillips, Mrs A. Creemer.

Pensby, Wirral. Dr E. M. Rule, Mrs M. F. Couche.

Pill, Avon. Dr K. M. Townend, Mrs V. Hawkins.

Pinhoe, Exeter, Devon. Dr R. Keith, Mrs M. Downes.

Potton, Bedfordshire. Dr B. M. Jones, Mrs H. Jones.

Radcliffe on Trent, Nottinghamshire. Dr G. S. Ripley, Dr M. Clamp, Mrs S. Ramsden.

Romsey, Hampshire. Dr C. Grant, Mrs J. Hayes, Mrs L. Matthews.

Rugby, Warwickshire. Dr D. Galliford, Mrs S. Barlow.

Runcorn, Cheshire. Dr I. G. Edwards, Mrs J. Toft.

Runcorn, Cheshire. Dr J. A. Newey, Mrs P. Skovgaard.

St Andrews, Fyfe. Dr H. A. Tait, Mrs B. Scott.

Salford, Greater Manchester. Dr J. W. Ferguson, Mrs P. Murray.

Sandy, Bedfordshire. Dr D. G. Milner, Dr A. Kapur, Mrs E. Millington.

Sawtrey, Huntingdonshire. Dr B. Dansie, Mrs A. Newell.

Selly Oak, Birmingham. Dr J. F. Harrison and Dr D. Cresswell, Dr R. Davis, Dr N. A. Duncan, Dr D. Fleming, Dr D. J. Handford, Dr J. Matthias, Dr K. G. Poyner, Dr J. Waters, Dr J. Watt.

Sheffield, Yorkshire. Dr M. P. Walsh, Mrs M. Robertson, Mrs H. McNamara.

Shipley, Yorkshire. Dr K. Haywood, Mrs N. Haywood.

Shipley, Yorkshire. Dr G. K. Renwick, Mrs A. Miller.

Shipley, Yorkshire. Dr I. Waite, Mrs M. Morrell.

Shipston-on-Stour, Warwickshire. The late Dr B. C. Smith, Dr T. F. C. Schofield, Mrs Y. Shepard, Mrs N. Wright.

Sleaford, Lincolnshire. Dr J. D. Collinge, Mrs D. Dowell, Mrs P. Walker.

Small Health, West Midlands. Dr R. G. Harrison, Mrs R. Ray.

Stantonbury, Milton Keynes. Dr P. Khurana, Dr P. K. Jayaram, Mrs K. Jones, Mrs F. Wright.

Stevenage, Hertfordshire. Dr D. H. R. Salter, Mrs C. Salter.

Stewarton, Ayrshire. Dr K. Hambly, Mrs M. Cheales.

Stockton on Tees, Cleveland. The late Dr H. C. Bergman, Dr A. McKenna, Mrs C. Groves, Mrs J. Armstrong.

Stratford-upon-Avon, Warwickshire. Dr M. H. F. Coigley, Mrs G. R. Barnes.

Stratford-upon-Avon, Warwickshire. Dr H. Nicol, Dr R. Peer, Miss M. Lumley, Mrs K. Marcus.

Stratford-upon-Avon, Warwickshire. Dr R. J. Fitchford, Mrs M. Sykes.

Stoke on Trent, Staffordshire. Dr D. F. Ferrington, Mrs J. Oakley.

Street, Somerset. Dr R. D. Last, Mrs S. Spearing.

Sutton in Ashfield, Nottinghamshire. Dr G. Stein, Mrs F. Stein, Mrs R. Irving.

Syston, Leicestershire. Dr M. G. F. Crowe, Mrs A. Crowe.

Thamesmead, London. Professor P. M. Higgins, Mrs D. S. Harding.

Todmorden, Lancashire. Dr J. M. S. Grieve, Mrs M. Houldsworth.

Tutbury, Staffordshire. Dr R. G. Spencer-Jones, Mrs C. Dalton.

Twickenham, Surrey. Dr G. Cassells-Brown, Mrs J. Cowley.

Wallasey, Merseyside. Dr N. A. Bradley, Dr S. C. Shah, Mrs C. Burns.

Watford, Hertfordshire. Dr R. G. Gain, Mrs M. Delaloye.

Watford, Hertfordshire. Dr P. Meager, Mrs P. Williams.

Wellesbourne, Warwickshire. Dr P. Gilbert, Miss M. Lumley.

Wellingborough, Northamptonshire. Dr I. F. Wall, Mrs B. Duncan.

Whitehaven, Cumbria. Dr R. H. Pearson, Mrs D. Connor, Mrs H. Whitehead.

Whitstable, Kent. Dr N. C. Macmillan, Sister P. J. Godding, Mrs L. Doyle.

Wideopen, Northumberland. Dr T. M. McKenzie, Mrs C. Beldon, Miss M. Armstrong.

Willesborough, Kent. Dr D. Sapsford, Miss E. Ellen.

Winchester, Hampshire. Dr C. Jenkins, Mrs B. Sworn.

Windermere, Cumbria. Dr J. A. Farndale, Mrs B. Davies, Mrs S. Miles.

Woodley, Berkshire. Dr M. A. Beale, Miss M. Roberts.

Woolpit, Suffolk. Dr N. Phillips, Mrs B. Scroxton.

Workington, Cumbria. Dr P. D. Burgul, Mrs M. Watson.

Worksop, Nottinghamshire. Dr W. J. Isherwood, Dr G. Moodie, Mrs S. Harrington.

Worthing, West Sussex. Dr A. J. Cairns, Mrs E. Crouch, Mrs S. Axtell.

Yaxley, Cambridgeshire. Dr C. R. Hart, Miss O. M. Holloway.

Screening Organisations

Bristol, Avon AHA Community Medicine Dept. Dr C. J. Burns-Cox, Dr D. Bainton, Mrs H. O. Watts.

BUPA, Pentonville Rd, London. Dr A. Bailey, Nurse B. Cundy.

Glasgow Blood Pressure Clinic, Western Infirmary, Glasgow. Dr A. Balmforth, Dr A. McKay, Dr H. A. Wapshaw, Sister I. Brown.

Glasgow Mass Radiography Service. Dr G. M. Stewart, Mrs J. Young.

Medical Research Council Blood Pressure Unit, Western Infirmary Glasgow. Dr G. Beevers, Dr P. L. Padfield, Dr R. Lever, Mrs J. Young.

Industrial Medical Centres

General Post Office, Leeds. Dr A. Hollingworth, Dr R. Davies, Mrs A. Butler.

General Post Office, Newcastle upon Tyne. Dr F. Turnbridge, Dr H. Ive, Mrs M. Grant.

General Post Office and British Telecom, Manchester, Dr J. Broxton, Dr A. Trimm, Mrs D. Jolley, Mrs M. Tasker.

Imperial Chemical Industries Pharmaceutical Division, Alderley Park. Dr G. W. Edward, Sister D. J. Bird.

Imperial Chemical Industries Pharmaceutical Division, Hurdsfield. Dr J. D. Broadbent, Sister K. Brown.

Imperial Chemical Industries Agricultural Division, Billingham. Dr B. K. B. Bain, Mrs B. S. Hebbron.

Imperial Chemical Industries Organics Division, Huddersfield. Dr A. J. M. Slovak, Dr G. H. Shaw.

Pilkington Bros, St Helens. Dr D. Jones, Mrs A. Derham, Mrs M. Pinnington.

1 Introduction

This is an account of an experiment. As medical experiments go it was a large and expensive one. It required the collaboration of several hundred doctors and nurses throughout the country and the participation of over half a million of their patients in a screening programme. Seventeen thousand of these patients agreed to take part in the full study, thereby committing themselves to taking tablets daily for over five years.

Medical research is almost always interesting to those who conduct it. This experiment was not only interesting but fun for those who carried out the work. Whether 'fun' would be an accurate description of the study from the point of view of the 17 000 participants is more debatable, but feedback (from those who felt sufficiently strongly to make their views known) was almost invariably favourable.

This particular medical experiment started with one real advantage. The question it was designed to answer was of major importance in medical practice and concerned a condition which contributed, perhaps more than any other, to cardiovascular morbidity and mortality in the United Kingdom. The question concerned the efficacy of treatment for mild hypertension – a disorder which affects millions of people throughout the world.

Epidemiological data and insurance statistics show steadily increasing risks with each increment of systolic or diastolic pressure starting from levels well within the range which is accepted as normal. There is no critical level of either pressure at which there is any sudden increase in morbidity or mortality (Fig. 1.1). Nor was there, in 1970, any reliable evidence that treatment did more good than harm within the range of pressures which would be considered as mild hypertension.

In 1970, the Medical Research Council was approached by a group of clinicians interested in the treatment of hypertension who proposed that a multicentre clinical trial should be carried out in patients with mild hypertension, in a hospital setting. At the same time the MRC received advice from its General Epidemiology Committee concerning the importance of investigating the value of treating mild hypertension in the community.

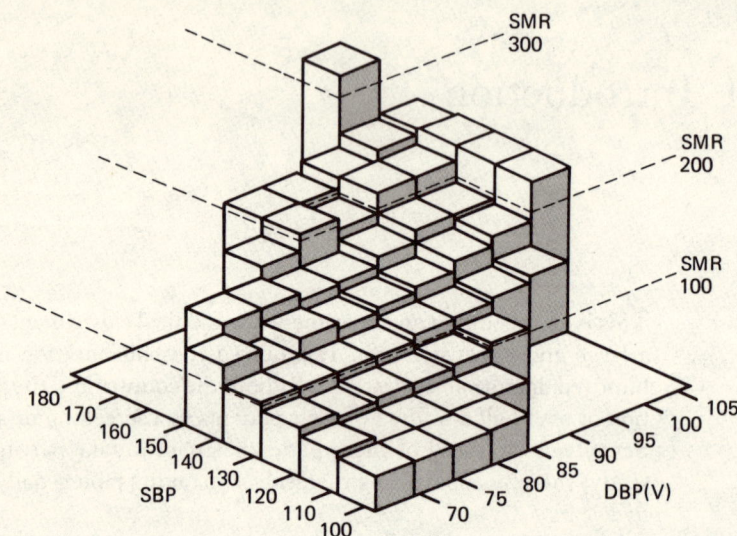

Fig. 1.1. *All-causes mortality, expressed as standardised mortality ratios, accord-ing to systolic and diastolic pressures. Data for men aged 40–69 years when accepted for insurance. Adapted from the US Society of Actuaries Blood Pressure Study, 1979.*

As a result the MRC appointed an ad hoc group 'to discuss the desirability and feasibility of a multicentre controlled trial in the treatment of mild to moderate hypertension, and if required to decide how this should be carried out and to advise the Council accordingly'. The group met several times that year. It recommended that the Council should go ahead with its own trial in the UK. The recommen-dation was accepted, and the ad hoc committee became an MRC Working Party, with a brief to plan and conduct a pilot trial. The pilot was started in 1973 and led on to the full-scale study which began in 1977 and finished in 1985.

In its way the MRC trial was a landmark in medical research in Britain. It showed, for the first time, the value of a highly motivated group of general practitioners who were willing to follow a protocol and accept the discipline necessary to keep to the rules required in any study of this kind. Professor (later Sir) Stanley Peart chaired the MRC Working Party from the days when it was an ad hoc committee to completion of the trial. He wrote that in his view the demonstration that a team of busy general practitioners could successfully carry out a research project of this size and complexity was more important than demonstrating whether or not it was of value to treat people with mild hypertension (Peart, 1980).

Be that as it may, this general practice research framework was a success and will continue to be useful for the kind of project which requires the co-operation of large numbers of the general population. Its success was partly attributable to the role played by nurses. This developed naturally as the trial progressed, and is described in detail later. The nurses were mostly part-timers who were appointed by the practices specifically for the trial work. They were keen, intelligent and enthusiastic and, because they usually had no other professional commitments, took charge of the day-to-day running of trial clinics and made them both efficient and friendly.

Throughout the trial the MRC Working Party took the scientific decisions but delegated the responsibility for the conduct of the trial to a Co-ordinating Centre in the MRC Epidemiology and Medical Care Unit at Northwick Park Hospital, Harrow. Three other committees were also involved. The so-called 'Systems Board' of the Council – (the Physiological Systems and Disorders Board) – was responsible for approving the study and for funding it. A Monitoring Committee (under the Chairmanship of Professor Geoffrey Rose) regularly reviewed the data concerning trial terminating events and provided reports for the independent Ethical Committee (under the Chairmanship of Sir Richard Doll) which was responsible for advising when the trial should stop. The parts played by these committees are described later; their interrelationships and lines of communication are illustrated in Fig. 1.2.

The aim of the trial was to give a 95% chance of detecting a 40% reduction in the number of deaths attributed to hypertension and in the number of fatal and non-fatal strokes, in people with mild hypertension given anti-hypertensive drugs when compared with a similar group not so treated. The difference was to be significant at the 1% level after 5 years follow-up of the participants. The participants were to be men and women aged 35–64 years with diastolic (phase V) pressures of 90–109 mm Hg.

It was obviously necessary that the treatment should be of a kind which could reasonably be available to patients cared for in general practice within the NHS. Results obtained using a system of medical care not widely available in the UK would have been of limited relevance: mild hypertension is such a common disorder that, if any recommendation about drug treatment were eventually to be made, this treatment and the system of patient management would need to be of a kind which general practitioners could reasonably hope to provide without disruption of their other work. This consideration made it appropriate to base the study mainly in general practices, although some industrial clinics and screening organisations were also involved. There was also a need to use readily available and safe drugs,

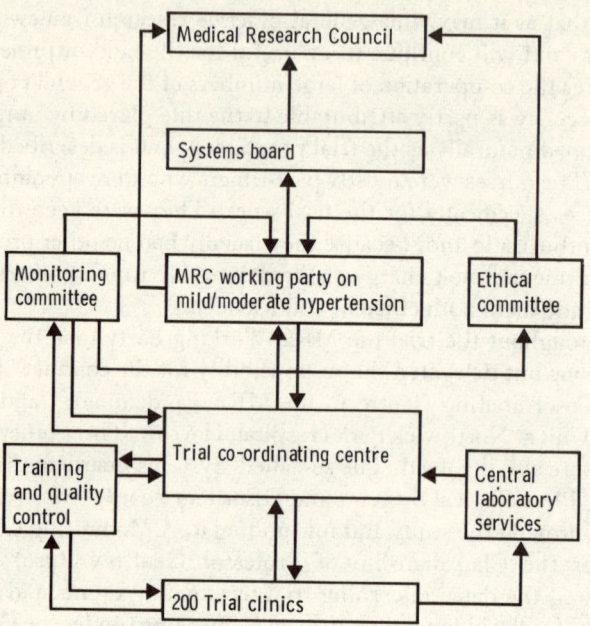

Fig. 1.2. *The structure of the trial.*

and from an early stage of the planning it seemed wise to build into the
study a comparison of thiazide diuretics and beta-adrenergic blocking
agents which had obvious metabolic and pharmacological differences
and offered scope for producing differences in respect of heart attacks
– the largest cause of morbidity and mortality.

   None of those who were in charge of the study had previous
experience of conducting a large therapeutic trial. As the trial progressed an unexpectedly large number of problems arose. Some could
be solved by incorporating sub-studies into the main trial. One such
sub-study was organised to determine whether bendrofluazide, which
formed one arm of the trial's treatment regime, was causing a high
prevalence of cardiac arrhythmias. Another was a study of the effects
on blood pressure and on serum biochemistry of two different doses of
the thiazide, with and without potassium supplements. The incor-
poration of these and other sub-studies into the work of the clinics
added interest to the normal trial routine and perhaps contributed to
the feeling, which became such a valuable feature of the organisation,
that the clinics were members of a large team.

   The study held an annual conference each year to which one nurse
and one doctor from each clinic were invited. These lively and
enjoyable two-day meetings also helped to unify the group. The

discussions at these meetings were remarkable not only for their quality but for the contributions made by the nurses. The almost fortuitous way in which the general practice research framework grew and particularly the way the nurses' role in it became so well integrated with that of the doctors, led to developments outside the remit of the trial but of considerable interest. A group of the trial practices, for example, got together and discussed and mounted so-called 'nurse-run hypertension clinics' for the hypertensive patients attending their practices but not in the trial. This was not an original thought, of course, but the idea of encouraging nurses to take a more active part in the management of hypertension certainly received some impetus from the success they had made of organising and running trial clinics.

During the very prolonged course of the MRC trial, the results of four other major national trials of the treament of mild hypertension were published. These were the US Public Health Service Study (USPHS), the Australian National Blood Pressure Study (ANBPS), the US Hypertension Detection and Follow-up Program (HDFP), and the Oslo trial. All four suggested that treatment reduced cerebro-vascular complications (WHO/ISH Mild Hypertension Liaison Committee, 1982). Some people believed that these other trials had pre-empted the British trial, but this view was not taken by the Working Party. There were difficulties about accepting the results of the American HDFP as relevant to the problem in Britain, and the results of the other studies were either inconclusive or, as was the case with the Australian trial, only at the margins of statistical significance. This is discussed in detail in Chapter 13. The questions which the MRC trial was designed to address had certainly not been satisfactorily answered from the point of view of the practising physician in Britain, so the trial was continued.

As it turned out it needed to be continued beyond the time when it had confirmed that treatment conferred a reduction in stroke inci-dence; this was partly because overall mortality in those on active treatment was, at that time, higher than that among untreated control subjects. As a result the trial accumulated data from over 85 000 person-years of observation and provided more opportunity for assessing the outcome in sub-groups of the population than had been possible in the other studies. It also provided more data on the costs as well as on the benefits of drug treatment for mild hypertension.

2 The pilot trial

The value of mounting a pilot trial before embarking on a full-scale study of the size and complexity of the MRC trial can hardly be exaggerated. There was much uncertainty about its feasibility, and particularly about the willingness of symptomless people to accept prolonged treatment with drugs which cause adverse reactions in some. Little was known about the prevalence of mild hypertension which would be found when the diagnosis was based on the number of measurements adopted for the screening programme, nor was it known what proportion of those eligible to enter the trial would agree to do so. This information was needed to estimate the total numbers to be screened, and the number of clinics to be recruited.

The first aim of the pilot trial was to recruit from 500 to 1000 adults aged between 35 and 64 years with blood pressures within the trial range (average diastolic phase V pressure of 90–109 mm Hg) and to follow them up in the trial for a period of two years. This would allow some idea of drop-out rates, of compliance with tablet-taking, of the incidence of adverse reactions to drugs administered, and of the adequacy of blood pressure control. Another aim was to measure the cost and efficiency of running the trial in different types of clinic, and thus be in a position to budget for the main study.

Other important objectives of the pilot trial were to develop reliable methods for carrying out the practical procedures involved, and to measure whether harm was being done to trial participants. In particular we were concerned that those who were previously asymptomatic and ignorant of their hypertension were not made neurotic by being told of their raised blood pressures and by being encouraged to allow themselves to be treated as patients.

Selection of collaborating centres

Twenty-five centres eventually collaborated in the pilot phase which started early in 1973. The authorisation of the main study was not made until the end of 1977 but once it was known that the main trial would be feasible, the pilot trial was allowed to expand beyond the numbers originally anticipated and to merge with the main trial. Since the pilot was large we intended, if possible, to incorporate its findings in the main trial analysis. It was not large enough, however, to check whether the estimated event rates were realistic.

The 25 centres were selected to cover a wide cross-section of medical practice but largely avoiding hospital clinics. Eleven were general practice groups, nine were industrial medical centres and five were linked with screening organisations.

General practices

The eleven centres involving general practice included practices of average list size about 10 000, and one group of such practices co-ordinated by a hospital consultant. Two were urban practices in large towns and two were in health centres in new urban housing estates; there was one suburban practice in the London commuter belt; three were practices based in market towns and two were in rural areas.

There were too few of these pilot trial clinics to provide anything more than impressions, but it was soon realised that some kinds of clinics were going to be more successful than others. Practices in large conurbations seemed less successful than those in smaller towns perhaps because they had a quicker than average turnover of both patients and doctors. Health centres dealing largely with the young and mobile populations of new housing estates were also less valuable to the trial. Large practices did not necessarily produce the expected numbers of patients for the trial perhaps because they could provide more cases than the doctors or nurses believed could be fitted into a manageable clinic. These impressions were subsequently confirmed in the main trial.

Following the pilot trial experience we aimed to recruit enthusiastic practices in small country towns where most of the inhabitants knew the four or five partners concerned. The eventual composition of the group of trial participants was probably biased by this type of selection, in favour of middle-class people registered with well organised practices. But the need for a fully representative population was considered less important than that the trial should be well conducted.

Industrial medical centres

The group of industrial medical centres included four clinics attached to large post office or telecommunications departments and five factory medical centres – two in the pharmaceutical industry and three in other manufacturing industries.

Two difficulties arose in connection with the use of industrial clinics. First, there are few industrial populations in Britain which have a work force in one area large enough to provide 100 mildly hypertensive subjects. Secondly, in times of economic constraint, industries are not keen to take on additonal work loads. Many industries were approached; few felt able to collaborate. Another lesson learnt at this stage was that the work force of the pharmaceutical industry, especially that involving research chemists, is both too introspective and too much in demand to be suitable for involvement in a study of this nature.

Screening organisations

Five clinics were based on screening organisations. Two of them were run in close collaboration with well organised screening programmes and presented few problems. Another linked with the pilot phase of a community screening programme was never adequately funded. One involved volunteers from management grades in business life and was therefore impossible to relate to any defined population. The fifth was based on hospital screening in 5 large teaching hospitals in a northern city, and recruited participants showing evidence of the sort of selection which occurs in hospital populations.

Decision to base the trial largely in general practice

The Working Party had recognised that general practitioners were always likely to be responsible for the detection and treatment of mild hypertension. It was therefore important that the effectiveness – or otherwise – of treatment should be demonstrated in the context of the type of care available in general practices in the National Health Service, and for this reason we were keen that the trial should be seen to be dealing with a representative sample of the general population (albeit from selected practices). This could be achieved only if the screening was conducted in properly defined populations (hence the need for age/sex registers) and obtained high response rates.

When the time came to enlarge the trial to its full size the decision to expand entirely in general practice was to some extent dictated by circumstances because, at that time, the climate in industry was unfavourable for involvement on the necessary scale and few screening programmes were available to join the trial. But in terms of both the practicability of the study and the applicability of the results to the general population of the United Kingdom, the decision seemed wise at the time and has certainly not been regretted since.

The practicability of trial procedures

At first we expected the doctors would carry out the trial work with the help of locally available staff. The MRC would pay for additional hours worked by nurses and secretaries but not by doctors. Administrators in the Department of Health and Social Security felt that paying doctors to carry out research on their own patients would set a precedent that the Department would be loath to follow. In fact the precedent had been set previously. General practitioners were already being remunerated for their part in other research programmes.

Detailed arrangements were left to the individual centres but had to include screening by a specially trained nurse. This required working from lists of the defined populations – age/sex registers in the case of general practices, pay-rolls in the case of industrial clinics, and the census tracts used by screening organisations where available. If a practice had no age/sex register the MRC covered the costs of compiling one.

In these early days of the pilot trial the whole programme of screening was slow and inefficient. Two innovations were largely responsible for improving the procedure. First, the age/sex registers were transferred to the computer at the Co-ordinating Centre, which allowed the rapid production of print-out lists and computer labels, and reduced the secretarial load to easily manageable proportions. Second, Merck, Sharp & Dohme Ltd donated a specially made mobile screening van. This could be parked in the practice car park or at some other convenient site, and had sufficient space for two patients to have their blood pressures taken simultaneously in individual cubicles, while others waited for a few minutes before their turn.

Initially, when a nurse had to arrange screening appointments, the despatch of screening invitation letters, and the running of screening clinics, all within the practice or medical centre premises, it had sometimes taken over a year to screen the 35–64-year-old members of a 10 000 practice list (Fig. 2.1). During this time, too, the work load was increasing as those who had been found suitable entered the trial and required regular follow-up. Computing the lists, and using mobile caravans, reduced the screening time to less than a month.

The importance of standardised measurements and clearly

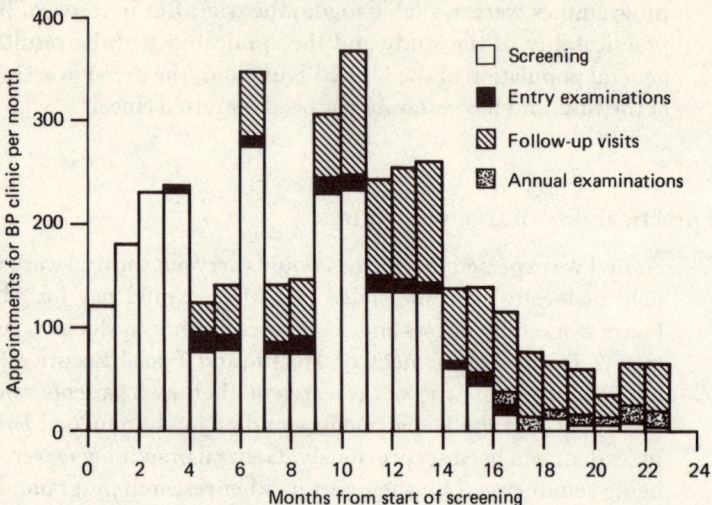

Fig. 2.1. *The load imposed by the trial on a group practice of list size 10 000 before computerised age/sex register and mobile screening facilities were made available.*

described clinical definitions and procedures had been recognised from the outset. A trial protocol and an operating manual (see Appendix) were provided for the use of doctors and nurses in each clinic. Printed cards for recording screening measurements (Fig. 2.2) and printed record booklets (Fig. 2.3) for the recording of clinical data were provided by the co-ordinating centre and proved satisfactory, though they required minor modifications as the trial progressed. The MRC also provided, on loan, two random-zero sphygmomanometers and a centrifuge for each clinic, sometimes an electrocardiograph and, if necessary, filing cabinets and drug cupboards. Initial supplies of labelled tablet containers were dispatched from the co-ordinating centre, stored at the clinic and replenished as necessary. The co-ordinating centre also provided a business reply service for correspondence with the co-ordinating centre, and for sending specimens (in specially designed packs, Fig. 2.4) to the Wolfson Research Laboratories in Birmingham.

As the pilot trial grew, however, it became obvious that a better organised system of training the staff at new clinics was needed and much more satisfactory arrangments, described in Chapter 3, led to a standardised approach which improved the efficiency of the clinics and the quality of the data they provided.

MRC TREATMENT TRIAL FOR MILD HYPERTENSION
BLOOD PRESSURE SCREENING

DATE .... CLINIC No. [|] 1,2

PATIENT'S SURNAME ....

Other Names ....

Address ....

....

Date of Birth .... Age ... ... [|] 3,4

OBSERVER'S CODE [|]   Sex ,.. ... ... [F] 5

PRACTITIONER'S NAME ....

Does the patient suffer from diabetes, asthma, gout,
    any other serious disease, or is the patient
    already on treatment for hypertension?
                        (Y=Yes N=No) ... [ ] 6

    If 'Yes', state which ....

Any other reason why patient is known
    to be unsuitable for screening? (Y=Yes N=No) ... [ ] 7

    If 'Yes', state reason ....

BLOOD PRESSURE READINGS I

	1	2	
Systolic	[| |]	[| |]	8–13
Diastolic	[| |]	[| |]	14–19
Zero Error	[ ]	[ ]	20–23
True Systolic	[| |]	[| |]	
True Diastolic	[| |]	[| |]	
True Systolic Mean	[| |]		
True Diastolic Mean	[| |]		

Date of next appointment ....

Fig. 2.2(a). *Blood pressure screening; record card. Side 1.*

BLOOD PRESSURE READINGS II

DATE .... OBSERVER'S CODE [|] 24,25

READINGS:-	1	2	
Systolic	[| |]	[| |]	26-31
Diastolic	[| |]	[| |]	32-37
Zero Error	[|]	[|]	38-41
True Systolic ...	[| |]	[| |]	
True Diastolic ...	[| |]	[| |]	
True Systolic Mean	[| |]		
True Diastolic Mean	[| |]		
GRAND SYSTOLIC MEAN (I + II/2)	[| |]		
GRAND DIASTOLIC MEAN (I + II/2)	[| |]		

Is patient suitable for entry examination?
(Y=Yes N=No) ... [ ] 42

If 'No', state reason ....

If 'Yes', insert date for
clinical examination ....

TO BE COMPLETED AFTER CLINICAL EXAMINATION

Has the patient been entered into trial?
(Y=Yes N=No) ... [ ] 43

If 'No', state reason ....

Fig. 2.2(b). *Blood pressure screening; record card. Side 2.*

CONFIDENTIAL   MRC TREATMENT TRIAL FOR MILD HYPERTENSION

ANNUAL EXAMINATION FORM

NAME   NUMBER [ ][ ][ ][ ][ ][ ][ ][ ] ,1-10
                                               Centre Age Sex Trial No. Letter Card No.

DATE OF EXAMINATION [ ][ ][ ] 11-16	PHYSICAL EXAMINATION		
Day Month Year	Body Weight		
MEDICAL HISTORY SINCE PREVIOUS ANNUAL EXAMINATION	(no shoes or jacket) Kg [ ][ ] 45-47		
(Please code answers Yes=Y No=N Doubtful=D and give further details if necessary in Section X)	st & lb [ ][ ] 48-51		
Heart disease			
Angina pectoris? Y, N or D [ ] 19	Cardiac rhythm Regular=R Irregular=I [ ] 52		
Myocardial infarction? Y, N or D [ ] 20	Cardiac murmurs/abnormal sounds? Y, N or D [ ] 53		
Congestive failure or cardiac asthma? Y, N or D [ ] 21	If 'Yes', specify		
Other heart disorder? Y or N [ ] 22	Evidence of cardiac failure? Y, N or D [ ] 54		
	If 'Yes', specify		
Peripheral artery disease			
Intermittent claudication? Y, N or D [ ] 23	CNS Signs? Y, N or D [ ] 55		
CNS	If 'Yes', specify		
Cerebrovascular episode? (transient ischaemic attack, hypertensive encephalopathy, stroke) Y, N or D [ ] 24	Fundi (Normal=N Grade I=1 Grade II=2 Grade III or more=3 Doubtful=D Unexamined=U) [ ] 56		
Other CNS Symptoms? (vision, balance sensory or motor disturbance &c) Y, N or D [ ] 25	INVESTIGATIONS		
Psychiatric disorder? Y, N or D [ ] 26	Electrocardiogram taken? Y or N [ ] 57		
Renal disease	Interpretation Normal=N Abnormal=A [ ] 58		
Nephritis, pyelonephritis, pyelitis, renal colic, haematuria, etc? Y, N or D [ ] 27	If abnormal, specify		
Respiratory disease	....		
Bronchial asthma? Y, N or D [ ] 28	Minnesota code reading		
Chronic Bronchitis? Y, N or D [ ] 29	I II III IV V VI VII VIII IX [ ][ ][ ][ ][ ][ ][ ][ ][ ] 59-67		
Other? Y or N [ ] 30	If coded VIII$_1$, specify Supraventricular=S Ventricular=V [ ] 68		
Alimentary system	Chest radiograph taken? Y or N [ ] 69		
Peptic ulcer? Y, N or D [ ] 31	Transverse cardiac diameter (mm) [ ][ ][ ] 70-72		
Constipation? Y, N or D [ ] 32	Transverse thoracic diameter (mm) [ ][ ][ ] 73-75		
Diarrhoea? Y, N or D [ ] 33	Urine Protein Negative=N Trace=T Positive=P Unknown=U [ ] 76		
Other? Y or N [ ] 34	Glucose Negative=N Light=L Medium=M Dark=D Unknown=U [ ] 77		
Metabolic and endocrine systems	Blood Urea (m mol/l) [ ][ ]		
Diabetes? Y, N or D [ ] 35	Uric acid (μ mol/l) [ ][ ]		
Gout? Y, N or D [ ] 36	Potassium (m mol/l) [ ][ ]		
Other? Y or N [ ] 37	Sodium (m mol/l) [ ][ ]		
Musculo-skeletal system	Cholesterol (m mol/l) [ ][ ]		
Arthritis? Y, N or D [ ] 38			
Other? Y or N [ ] 39			
FOR FEMALES ONLY On the 'pill'? Y or N [ ] 41	Any reason now for withdrawing from randomised treatment? Y or N [ ] 78		
SMOKING Cigarettes smoked now? Y or N [ ] 42	If 'Yes', please complete 'Withdrawal from randomised treatment' form		
If 'Yes', how many per day? [ ][ ] 43,44	COMMENTS		
SECTION X Insert any further details relevant to history and symptoms here			
....			
....			
....	Signed		

Fig. 2.3. *Record booklet for clinical follow-up data – a sample page.*

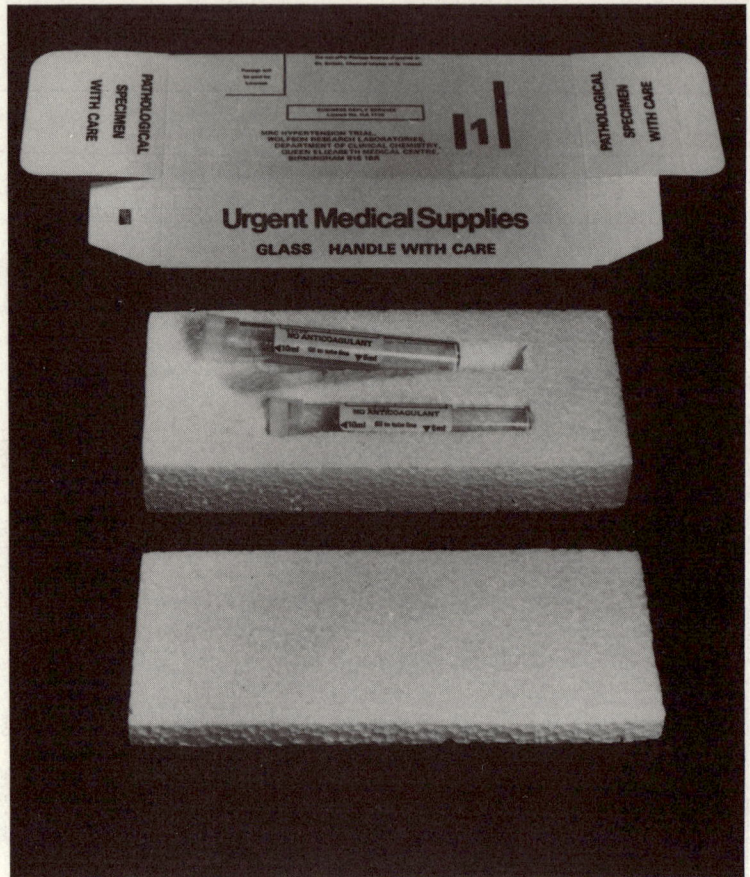

Fig. 2.4. *Postal pack for serological specimens.*

Criteria for entry to the trial

Blood pressure measurements were recorded twice, consecutively, after subjects had been sitting for at least 10 minutes, of which the last three had to be spent sitting where the measurements were made. For those in whom the mean of these two measurements equalled or exceeded 200 mm Hg systolic pressure, or 90 mm Hg diastolic (fifth phase), an appointment was made for a second examination. Others were reassured and dismissed. Two further readings were made for those recalled, usually one week but not more than 4 weeks after the first. Mean values of the four readings were calculated; if these were below 200 mm Hg systolic and below 90 mm Hg diastolic, the subjects were reassured; if equal to or above 200 mm Hg systolic or 110 mm Hg diastolic they were referred to their own GPs for investigation or

Table 2.1. *The grounds for exclusion from the trial*

1 Known underlying cause (secondary hypertension)
2 Anti-hypertensive therapy in last 3 months
3 Normally accepted indications for therapy (ophthalmic, renal or cardiac)
4 Myocardial infarction or stroke within last 3 months
5 Angina pectoris or intermittent claudication
6 Concurrent serious disease
7 Pregnancy, diabetes, gout or bronchial asthma
8 History of significant psychiatric disorder
9 Serum potassium of 3.4 mmol/l or less
10 Serum urea 8.3 mmol/l or more

treatment. If the mean of the 4 readings was within the trial range (a diastolic pressure of 90–109 mm Hg providing the systolic pressure was less than 200 mm Hg) an appointment was made for the pressure to be checked by a doctor.

Only when the doctor had confirmed that the screening readings were still in the trial range (after recall if necessary) did he or she explain the trial to the patient, allow an opportunity for questioning, and ask whether or not the patient was willing to participate. Those that agreed signed a consent form, as did their own general practitioners. Each person entering the trial did so, therefore, on the basis of six or eight blood pressure measurements taken over a period of 4 to 12 weeks.

By this stage the only screened subjects excluded were those whose blood pressures were outside the trial range, those who had received antihypertensive therapy within the preceding 3 months, those who had suffered a stroke or a myocardial infarction within the preceding 3 months and those with contraindications to taking either a thiazide diuretic or a beta-blocking drug. The remainder were called for an entry medical examination which consisted of taking a medical history, a physical examination including ophthalmoscopy, the meaurement of height and body weight, a 12-lead electrocardiogram (ECG) and urine and blood tests.

Providing no excluding conditions (Table 2.1) had been detected during this examination, the patient's name was recorded in the next available space on a computer print-out register comprised of 6 separate sheets (one for each of the three decades of age for the two sexes) which listed trial numbers, specific for each clinic. Against these numbers were printed, in random order but balanced every 8 numbers, four coded primary treatment regimes, 1, 2, 3 and 4. This open method of random allocation to groups receiving either of the two active tablets (Regimes 1 and 2, bendrofluazide and propranolol) or to groups receiving matching placebo tablets (Regimes 3 and 4) was simple, worked satisfactorily and without detectable abuse.

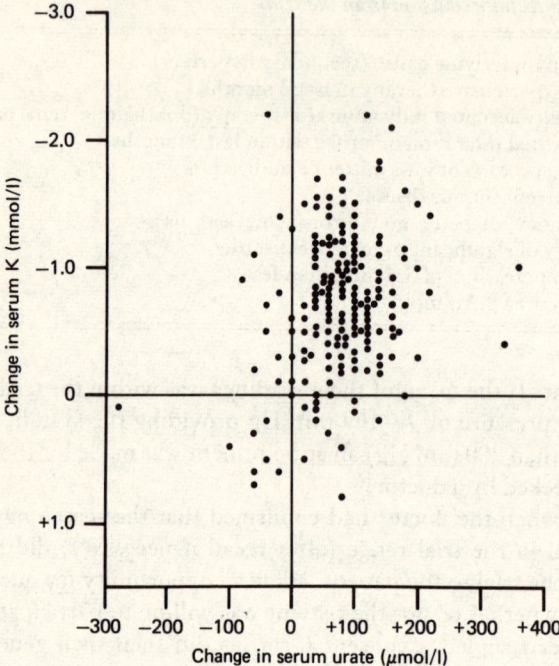

Fig. 2.5. *Changes in serum potassium and serum urate levels from entry to 1 year in those taking bendrofluazide (pilot trial data only).*

Pilot trial results

By February 1977, when the progress of the pilot phase was reported (Medical Research Council Working Party on Mild to Moderate Hypertension, 1977), 1849 people had entered the pilot trial (1092 men and 757 women); 972 had been under observation for more than 1 year, 629 for over 2 years, and 219 for over 3 years.

Among the general practices involved in the pilot trial, the response to the screening invitations varied between 65% and 90%; over 90% of those found eligible for the trial entered it. Compliance with medication seemed satisfactory as judged by tablet counts, by the biochemical response of those on bendrofluazide (Fig. 2.5) and by the pulse rate change in those on propranolol (Fig. 2.6). Three years after entry to the trial 82% were still under regular observation. The remaining 18% had either stopped of their own accord or on the wishes of their doctors, or had moved to areas far from a trial clinic, or had died.

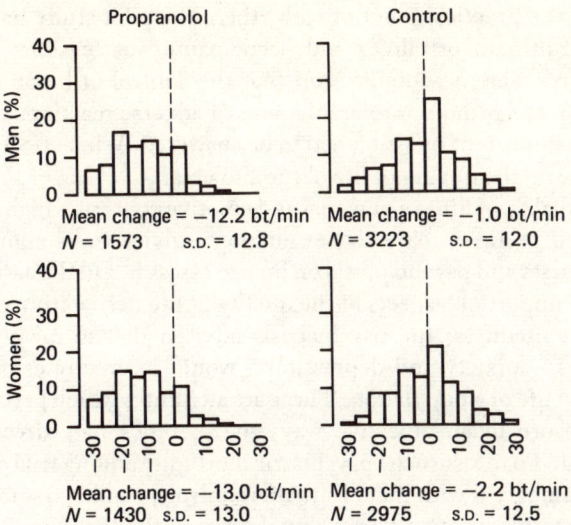

Fig. 2.6. *Changes in pulse rates (beats/min) from entry to 1 year in propranolol and control groups.*

The differences in mean pressure between treated and control subjects (13–17 mm Hg systolic and 6–8 mm Hg diastolic) were less than expected because the fall in the pressure among controls, after entry to the trial, was both greater and continued for longer than was anticipated. But the differences in the distributions of blood pressures of treated and control subjects, at one year after entry to the study, were used to re-estimate the numbers required for the full-scale study and confirmed that between 15 000 and 19 000 subjects would be needed. (Note: This re-estimate had to be based on the doubtful assumption that the rate of morbidity experienced by those treated would revert to that of subjects who had similar blood pressure levels without treatment.)

The acceptability of the trial procedures was assessed at screening, and at entry to the trial, by response rates and during the follow-up by compliance with tablet taking, by drop-out rates and, less quantitatively, from feed-back from clinics and patients. After $2\frac{1}{2}$ years in the pilot trial 21% of men and 9% of women on bendrofluazide and 8% of men and 15% of women on propranolol had stopped taking their allocated treatment because of adverse reactions. Most had been transferred from one active primary drug regime to the other and had continued treatment. Collaborating clinics welcomed the trial as an opportunity to deal systematically with the problem of hypertension in their practices; patients seemed to appreciate their doctors' participation in an investigation of preventive measures.

From the practical point of view, then, the pilot study had shown that recruitment of clinics and participants was feasible, that the procedures were acceptable, and that the control of blood pressure was adequate without intolerable rates of adverse reactions to drugs. Another important question had to be answered. What effects did the trial have on the quality of life of the subjects?

The quality of life is a personal and emotive concept which does not lend itself to direct, objective evaluation. Advice was sought among psychiatrists and psychologists on how to assess it. On the assumption that two important aspects of the quality of life derive from calmness and contentedness, the psychiatrists advised that to measure their opposites – anxiety and depression – would indirectly estimate the quality of life of a population. These are attributes which psychiatrists can measure in an objective way; the methods had already been validated. To measure the psychiatric morbidity among trial entrants, and to compare it with that of suitable controls, would go some way to answering the question posed. Furthermore, the Working Party was keen to be in a position to answer comments often made that any physical benefits resulting from early treatment of an asymptomatic condition might be bought at the expense of increased neurosis or anxiety. The proposed study would allow that reasonable concern to be confirmed or refuted on the basis of facts rather than impressions.

The study, carried out from the Institute of Psychiatry by Dr A. H. Mann, with advice from Professor Michael Shepherd, was devised to measure the effect on the participants of three features of the trial. These were:

(a) being told that the blood pressure was raised;
(b) having to attend a clinic regularly as a patient;
(c) taking antihypertensive medication, some of which was known to have psychotropic effects.

A method of screening for psychiatric morbidity on a large scale was required, and a suitable means of doing this was the two-stage system devised and validated by Goldberg (1972). This consists of the General Health Questionnaire (GHQ) followed by a Standard Psychiatric Interview to diagnose those who indicate by their response to the questionnaire that they are likely to be psychiatric cases (Goldberg *et al.*, 1970). These tests had been validated only as means of identifying what psychiatrists consider to be illnesses. This is not necessarily the same as anxiety in mentally healthy people; it is quite possible that the study would have failed to identify psychologically normal people (or their spouses) who lay awake at night thinking about the trial and its implications.

The design of the study is shown in Table 2.2. Subjects attending blood pressure screening centres were asked to complete the 30 item

Table 2.2. *The design of the psychiatric study*

Subjects (35–64 years) attending MRC clinics for blood pressure check (GHQ-A)

Result of B.P. check	Result of recall	Trial participants matched with controls for psychiatric study	3 month follow-up	1 year follow-up
Severely hypertensive D.B.P. below 90 mm Hg	Pressure below 90 mm Hg	Normal controls	Normal controls	Normal controls
For recall D.B.P. 90–109 mm Hg	Suitable for trial 90–109 mm Hg	Recalled controls Trial participants	Recalled controls Trial participants	Recalled controls Trial participants
		(B)	(C)	(D)
GHQ Psychiatric interview conducted		*	*	*

short form of the questionnaire (GHQ) before having their blood pressure measured. Those who subsequently entered the trial were matched by age, sex and response to the initial questionnaire (GHQ-A) with two controls. One control subject was selected at random from those who had been found to have normal blood pressure; a second control was selected at random from those who were recalled on account of their initially raised pressure but reassured at the next check.

At entry to the trial, each participant completed a second GHQ (GHQ-B), and as soon as possible thereafter the two matched controls also completed a second GHQ. This procedure was repeated at 3 months after entry (GHQ-C) and again one year after entry (GHQ-D). The detailed results of this study have been reported (Mann, 1977, 1984). It included 235 trial subjects and similar numbers in the two control groups.

Between screening (GHQ-A) and entry (GHQ-B) no significant differences in the incidence of new 'cases' (i.e. positive responders), or of 'cures' (i.e. changes from positive to negative response), were found between the 3 groups, indicating that informing asymptomatic people of their raised blood pressure caused no undue psychological disturbance. Between entry (GHQ-B) and 3 months after entry (GHQ-C) the prevalence of positive responders became significantly lower in trial participants than in normal controls ($P < 0.01$) and just significantly lower than in recalled controls ($P < 0.05$). The incidence of new positive responders did not differ significantly between the 3 groups. The change from positive to negative GHQ response was significantly greater in trial cases than in either control group. This indicated that participation in the trial did not cause psychological disturbance, and suggested that those who entered with psychological symptoms benefited from their contact with the clinic. Between entry (GHQ-B) and 1 year after entry (GHQ-D) the incidence of new cases between the 3 groups did not differ significantly but the change from positive to negative responses remained significantly greater in trial participants than in either control group. Interviews with a psychiatrist confirmed the results obtained from questionnaires.

It was concluded that the study (so far as it went) had shown no evidence of any adverse effect on the quality of life, as measured by the incidence of morbid anxiety and depression. If the antihypertensive treatment had caused symptoms of a physical nature these would have been revealed, and the pilot experience suggested that the adverse reactions were largely minor and reversible. This reassuring result came from the first published study of an attempt to measure the psychological effects of a screening programme on its participants.

The results of the pilot trial had therefore shown that a full-scale study was scientifically and ethically justified and administratively feasible. The next step was to estimate its costs.

Estimates of the costs for a full-scale trial

During the early phases of a pilot trial of this kind expenditure per subject is disproportionately high compared with the costs of following subjects in the later phases. In the MRC trial this was due to the relatively high expenditure on capital equipment, the preparation of age/sex registers, and on the screening and intensive follow-up in the early months. When allowance was made for this, and expenditure was extrapolated to cover a full 5 years of follow-up, it was estimated that the average cost of following one person for a year in the general practice clinics would amount to £23.50 (at 1976 prices).

At a cost of £23.50 per person-year the required 90 000 person-years of observation (18 000 subjects for 5 years) would result in expenditure of £2 115 000, less the costs (£81 000) already incurred on the pilot trial which would form part of the main study. Thus about £2 000 000 would be needed for the full-scale study, spread over a period of about 10 years allowing for initial expansion and final contraction. Annual expenditure was estimated to peak at something in excess of £300 000.

These estimates did not include the full costs of the co-ordinating centre, or the cost of trial drugs which were donated by the pharmaceutical companies, or the cost of the biochemical work which was independently financed. The actual costs incurred are discussed later. Naturally, they were influenced by inflation, but in recommending that the full-scale trial should go ahead the Working Party was conscious of the need to prune the costs and considered many ways of doing this.

The rigour of the statistical design, and the fact that it assumed no reduction in coronary heart disease from anti-hypertensive treatment, dictated the large numbers required. Calculations based on pilot trial data had suggested that about 17 500 subjects would be required for the design as suggested. If instead of a trial with a 95% chance of demonstrating a 40% reduction in the specified events, significant at the 1% level, using a 2-tailed test, certain modifications were introduced, they would diminish the estimated size of the trial as shown in Table 2.3. There were clearly opportunities for a cheaper package but the Working Party was unwilling to sacrifice robustness for expediency.

It was possible that some of the financial burden could be shared with other Western European countries willing to work to a similar

Table 2.3. *Numbers of individuals required for different
statistical designs*

Power (%)	Significance (%)	Test	Numbers required
95	1	1-tailed	15 510
90	1	2-tailed	14 624
95	5	2-tailed	12 782
90	5	1-tailed	8414

protocol. Attempts to encourage the mounting of compatible trials in other countries were made, but not successfully. In many Western European countries the pattern of primary care services prevents the study of defined populations and though hospital-based programmes would have been possible, the Working Party had deliberately tried to avoid the use of hospital populations in Britain.

One change which would markedly reduce the costs of screening would be to use several mobile screening units rather than the single one used in the pilot phase, and the Working Party recommended that this should be done. The costs for the main trial using mobile screening units, including the costs of the co-ordinating centre but excluding drugs and biochemical testing, were finally estimated at £2 034 000.

On the basis of these estimates and the results of the pilot trial the Systems Board recommended expansion to the full-scale study and the Council authorised this in July 1977.

3 The screening programme

The pilot phase of the trial had shown a prevalence of 4.7% of screened subjects suitable and willing to enter the study. Extrapolation from this indicated that about half a million people would need to be invited for screening to achieve 400 000 people screened which would enable the trial to reach its target of 18 000 participants. General practices with a total list of 10 000 were entering an average of 90 to 100 people; from this it seemed likely that 180 to 200 practices would need to be recruited.

Several different ways of recruiting clinics were tried. Indirect approaches were unsuccessful; letters encouraging Area Health Authorities and the administrators of Family Practitioner Committees to provide lists of suitable practices produced a small response, as did approaches through academic departments of General Practice. Talks by members of the Working Party at postgraduate medical meetings, a video tape for use at such meetings and in individual practices, and tape recordings were all used and presumably helped to get the trial well known, but achieved little direct response.

Letters to the correspondence columns of the medical journals and articles in general practitioner newspapers produced a larger number of useful enquiries but the most effective way of recruiting was by asking practices already collaborating to approach others. A loose-leaf letter written by participating general practitioners and inserted into the pages of the Journal of the Royal College of General Practitioners also stimulated a useful response from suitable practices. Perhaps somewhat surprisingly direct approaches through the Department of Health and the Royal College of General Practitioners were of little value.

Doctors who responded to any of the various approaches were sent more information about the study, about the additional work load which it imposed, and about the arrangements which the MRC could make to ensure that this was manageable. They were also sent a questionnaire which would provide the co-ordinating centre with more information about each practice – its size, the number of partners, whether there were branch surgeries and if so how many and how distant from the main surgery, whether the practice had an up-to-date age/sex register, an electrocardiograph and a centrifuge.

All practices which showed interest in the trial and appeared suitable in terms of size and location were visited by one of the two doctors at the co-ordinating centre. These visits, which usually involved a meeting with most of the partners and lasted about an hour, provided an opportunity for both parties to gain a better appreciation of the situation. The partners learnt more about the trial protocol, the procedures and the help which would be offered by the MRC. The co-ordinating centre was able to judge the enthusiasm of the practice and whether this was shared by most partners, the suitability of the practice accommodation as regards space, and the accessibility of the central surgery to patients who might normally attend branch surgeries. This was an important consideration in the running of follow-up clinics.

Only about 50% of the practices visited actually joined the study. Those that did not were about equally divided between practices which were unwilling to participate – often for the good reason that not all partners were in favour of involvement – and practices which for one reason or another were unsuitable.

Suitable practices were advised to contact, by telephone, others already in the trial to learn, at first-hand, about the pros and cons of joining the trial. Once the decision had been taken and the practice had found the right nurse to take on trial duties, a doctor and this nurse were encouraged to visit a trial training practice in Stratford-upon-Avon (Dr M. H. F. Coigley and Mrs Greta Barnes), at the MRC's expense, to discuss the setting up of a trial clinic. This was the first stage of a training programme which resulted in a welcome standardisation of methodology; it was also the first component of a programme which made the doctors and nurses involved in trial clinics realise that they were joining a large team working towards a common aim. One of the pleasing features of the trial, as it progressed, was the way morale remained high throughout its long duration despite the fact that each practice recognised that its own contribution was only a small part of the whole.

Screening methods

A choice of different screening methods was available. For group practices which had space in their car parks but little spare accommodation within the surgery, the use of one of the trial's mobile screening units enabled rapid screening to be undertaken with little disruption of practice routine. The screening caravans were purpose-

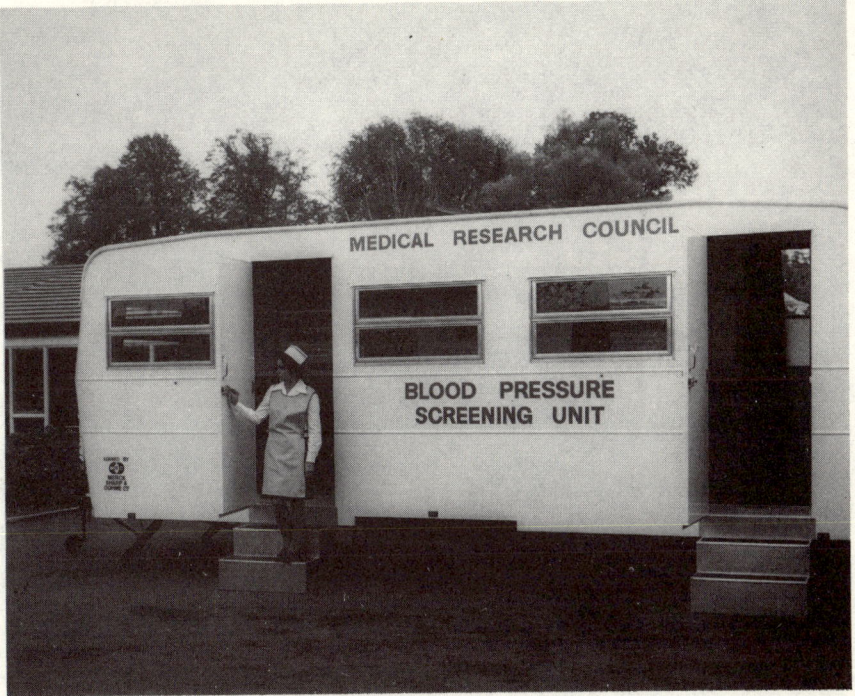

Fig. 3.1. *One of the purpose-built mobile screening caravans.*

built (or purpose-adapted). The trial owned one and rented five
others. They were the largest size of caravan permitted to be towed on
British roads – 22′ long and 7′ wide (Fig. 3.1). Each was divided
internally to provide a reception area, with a desk for the receptionist
and a seat where people sat for 10 minutes before having their blood
pressures recorded (Fig. 3.2). There were two cubicles for blood
pressure measurement (Fig. 3.3).

The screening caravans were staffed usually by a team of 6 state-
registered nurses – the trial nurse (who led the team) and 5 others. All
were locally recruited but trained by the trial's training nurses, and
their competence in recording accurate measurements was tested
before screening began. As they worked in two shifts, the van could be
kept open from 9.00 a.m. to 7.00 or 8.00 p.m., and the three nurses in
each shift rotated so that each in turn acted as receptionist while two
recorded blood pressures. With this technique, up to 200 people could
be screened daily and the screening of the 3 300 35–64-year-old people
found in a practice with a total list size of 10 000 would normally be
completed in about 20 working days.

About 10% of those screened required to be recalled because their
first blood pressure readings were elevated, and these recall visits were

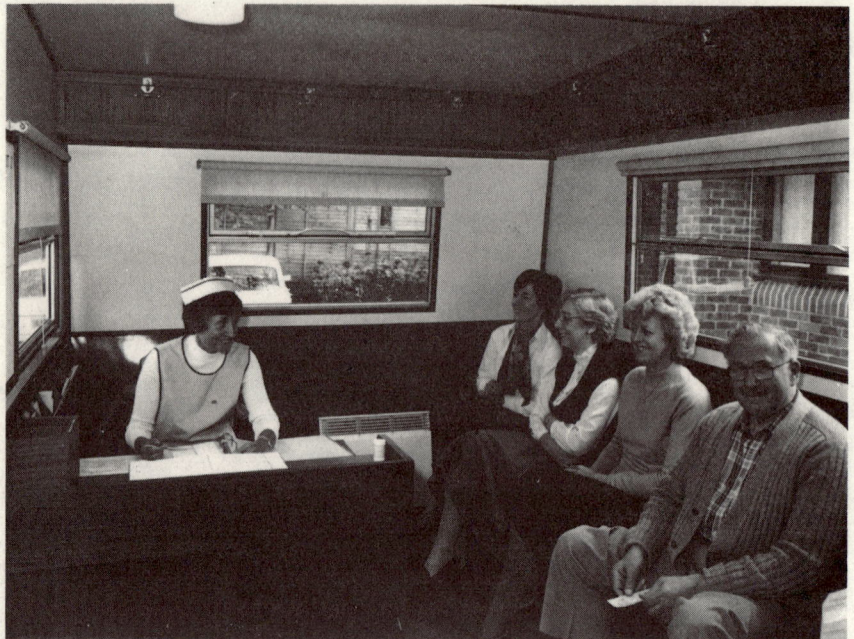

Fig. 3.2. *Reception for screening.*

fitted into the schedule for the screeners and took place in the caravan. Reminder postcards for those who had failed to respond to the first invitation were sent towards the end of the programme at each clinic. Although the screening was intended to cover only those sent invitation letters, inevitably others attended and were rarely refused examination; if hypertension was discovered their own GPs were notified of the findings by letter.

The programme for the screening vans operated to a pre-arranged schedule. Each caravan arrived at a practice complete with 4 sphygmomanometers – 2 of which were spare ones – and all the necessary stationery and screening cards. At the end of its visit to one practice the van was towed, by professionals, to the next site. The arrangements for this were made by the practices locally, and worked well. Once a year, or more often if needed, the caravans were serviced and restocked.

Of the 176 general practices which contributed to the study, 139 used mobile screening facilities.

If a practice had spare accommodation and could provide facilities equivalent to those in the caravans – a reception and waiting area and two rooms for blood pressure recording – the same type of rapid screening programme was mounted and 11 clinics conducted 'crash' screening programmes of this kind.

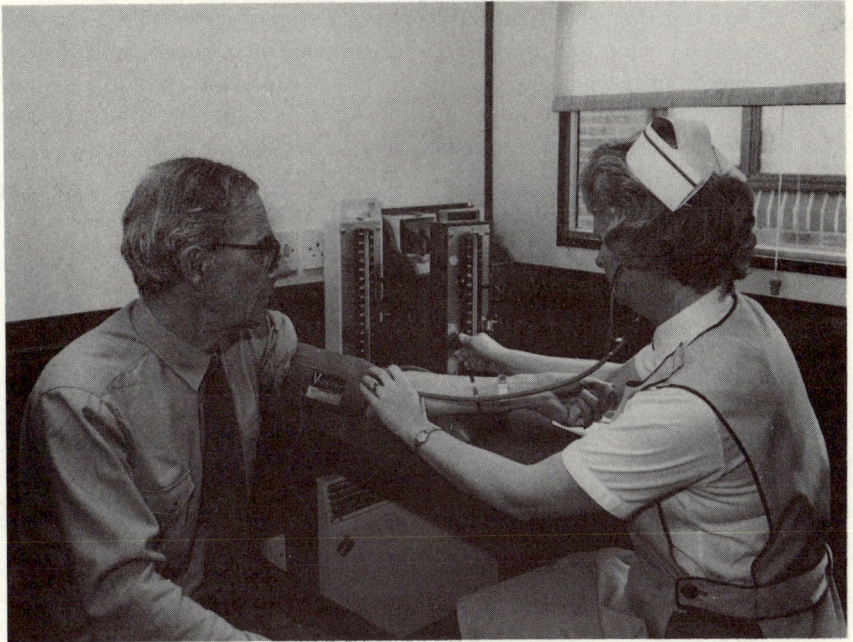

Fig. 3.3. *Blood pressure measurement at screening.*

The remaining 26 general practice clinics, including most of those recruited early in the trial, screened more slowly in their own accommodation with fewer staff. The 9 industrial medical centres used their own staff and facilities but used Random-Zero sphygmomanometers (Wright and Dore, 1964) provided by the trial and exactly followed the trial's screening methods, as did 3 of the 5 screening organisations which contributed to the trial. Two screening programmes which had already finished screening using the London School of Hygiene instrument (Rose, Holland and Crowley, 1964) before the decision to join the trial, had included only 45–64-year-old people and their methodology differed in minor respects from that adopted in other clinics.

The logistics of screening

Supplies of screening equipment were sent to each clinic to arrive one month before screening was scheduled to start. These included random-zero sphygmomanometers and instructions for their use and all stationery needed before eligible subjects were asked to attend for an entry medical examination.

Sufficient copies of a screening invitation letter, under the practice's letterhead, were duplicated at the co-ordinating centre and these were sent together with print-outs of the age/sex register for 35–64-year-old people, computer-produced labels, appointment sheets, information sheets for receptionists, advice on how to explain the trial to potential participants, and consent forms. Posters and suggestions for publicity – in local newspapers for example – were also sent to the clinics with these initial supplies.

The first task of the trial nurse was to prepare invitation letters with appointments. This was done using the computer print-out sheets which gave the names and addresses of all those in the age range. The lists were in alphabetical order of surname with both sexes on the same list; those with the same surname and address were listed adjacently. Appointment times were recorded on separate appointment sheets and written into the letters. Where addresses were the same for subjects with the same name – as, for example, man and wife – an economy on postage was made by including appointments for both on the same letter. The trial nurse worked through the entire list preparing all such invitation letters in advance, but the posting was staggered so that letters were dispatched only a week before the appointment was due. For the first 2 days of screening, clinics made appointments for about 2 patients every 5 minutes; thereafter they sent for 3 people every 5 minutes. In practice this meant inviting 150–200 people for each of the first two days, and 225–275 thereafter. These figures allowed for the 25% non-response which was usually found.

Three computer labels were provided for each person on the computer list. These were intended to streamline the clerical work. The first was used to address the envelope for the invitation letter; the second, for identification on the card used for recording screening measurements; the third, which had the blood pressure measurements recorded on it after screening, was stuck into the patient's NHS notes.

The screening went on every weekday and on Saturday mornings. The load was heaviest during the early evenings because those who could not conveniently keep their given appointments earlier in the day were encouraged to attend between (say) 5.30 and 7.30 p.m. For this reason no appointments were given for this period.

As people attended for screening their names were ticked off the computer list and they were handed a computer-labelled screening card and then sat waiting for 10 minutes to allow their blood pressures to settle. They were then questioned about conditions which would exclude them from the trial (such as treatment for hypertension, recent stroke or myocardial infarction, diabetes, gout, bronchial asthma, etc.) and this was recorded on the screening cards before they had two immediately consecutive recordings of their blood pressures.

```
        PATIENT'S SURNAME (Please Print) ..................

        PATIENT'S TRIAL NUMBER ...........................


            MRC TREATMENT TRIAL FOR MILD HYPERTENSION
                         CONSENT FORM

 It is possible that treatment might help people whose blood pressure is
 only mildly elevated above normal values.

 We are helping the Medical Research Council to conduct a trial to assess
 the need for treatment in such cases and your blood pressure has been
 found to be at a level where tablets might benefit you.

 All who are enrolled into the trial will be kept under regular medical
 supervision and will receive either one of several different kinds of
 tablet, some of which have no effect, or careful observation only.
 Anyone whose blood pressure is found to rise to levels where there is
 no doubt that treatment is beneficial would be withdrawn from the trial
 and given appropriate treatment.

 We would be grateful if you would sign the accompanying form if you are
 willing to enter the trial.  Obviously, you can withdraw at any stage
 if you wish.
 ──────────────────────────────────────────────────────────────────────

 I have read the above explanation and the nature of the trial has been
 explained orally to me and I have had an opportunity of asking any
 questions.  It is on the basis of the explanation and the information
 in this form that I agree to participate in the blood pressure treatment
 trial.

                              Signed ..............................

                              Date ...............................

 ──────────────────────────────────────────────────────────────────────

 Family physician's agreement

 I am the general practitioner of the above patient and in my opinion
 there is nothing in the medical history to contraindicate entry into
 the trial.  The patient would enter the trial with my consent.

                              Signed ..............................

                              Date ...............................
```

Fig. 3.4. *The form used for recording informed consent.*

Those with pressures below the trial range were reassured and thanked; those requiring recall were given an appointment card and requested to attend again in a week for two further blood pressure measurements.

Those whose mean pressures were still within the trial range after recall were given another appointment and this time the blood pressure was checked by a doctor, again using the random-zero sphygmomanometer. If the screening readings were again confirmed as within the trial's range (after further recall, if necessary) the doctor or nurse explained the trial in detail, gave an opportunity for questions and obtained written consent from both the patient and from his or her own family practitioner. The consent form is shown in Fig. 3.4.

Those who entered the trial therefore, did so on the basis of 6 or 8 measurements made on 3 or 4 separate occasions.

The training of screening methods

State registered nurses, who were recruited locally by the practice, were employed to help the trial nurse with the screening at each clinic. Instruction was given by one of the team of training nurses on the day before screening was due to start; the instruction covered three topics.

First the standardisation of blood pressure recording was done using the blood pressure training device described by Rose (1965). This comprised two series of tape recordings, each consisting of the Korotkov sounds of 12 subjects; the first series was used for training and the second for testing purposes. Before each recording was an announcement of subject identification followed by a time marker – '3, 2, 1 – start'. At 'start' two stop watches were set in motion. The first was stopped at the first appearance of systolic sounds, the second at the disappearance of sounds. For each recording the observer noted her estimate of systolic and diastolic (phase 5) pressure expressed as the time interval from the first time marker. After correcting, if necessary, for differences in tape-recorder speed the trainee observer could compare her own readings with standards. As all recordings were made with a constant deflation rate of 2 mm Hg per second, differences from standard readings could be expressed in terms of mm Hg. Once readings were standardised on the training tape, to give a mean time interval within one second (2 mm Hg) of the standard and with no large discrepancies on individual tracings, the trainee repeated the performance using the series of testing recordings, for which no list of standard timings was provided. Performances on the testing tape were checked by the training nurses. Perhaps the main value of this training was to make observers realise that careful accurate blood pressure observations were required and that inaccuracy could be detected objectively.

The second aim of the training was to familiarise nurses with the Hawksley Random-Zero sphygmomanometer. (Note: This instrument is made in two forms. The trial used instruments with zero-error ranges of 60 mm Hg.) This instrument is basically an orthodox mercury manometer in which the effective amount of mercury is varied between consecutive measurements in such a way that the observer is unaware, until after the reading has been recorded, of the size of the variation. The instrument incorporates an unusually tall mercury reservoir which communicates with both the manometer

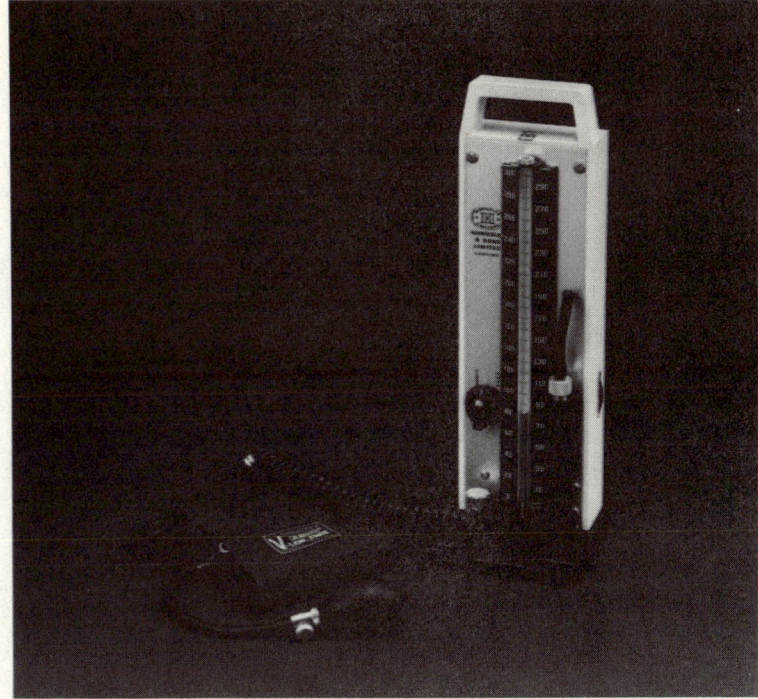

Fig. 3.5. *The Hawksley Random-Zero sphygmomanometer.*

and, via a tap, with an expansible reserve mercury chamber (Fig. 3.5). The capacity of this reserve chamber (Fig. 3.6) is determined by the position of a cam, controlled by a thumbwheel on the outside of the instrument. On inflation the manometer and the reserve chamber fill with mercury. When the reserve chamber is full the tap is switched to close off the mercury it contains. Manometer readings are then made in the usual way but a zero error, which varies according to the contents of the reserve chamber, has to be subtracted from each. The instrument therefore allows the recording of a series of consecutive but independent observations. A little extra time is needed for the subtraction of the zero error, and observers require some practice in the instrument's use. Having demonstrated the instrument and instructed the nurses how to use it, the training nurses tested the accuracy of their observations on a patient, this time using a training stethoscope with two sets of ear-pieces.

Finally, advice was given on the administrative aspects of screening, and instruction on the blood pressure criteria for the trial (Fig. 3.7).

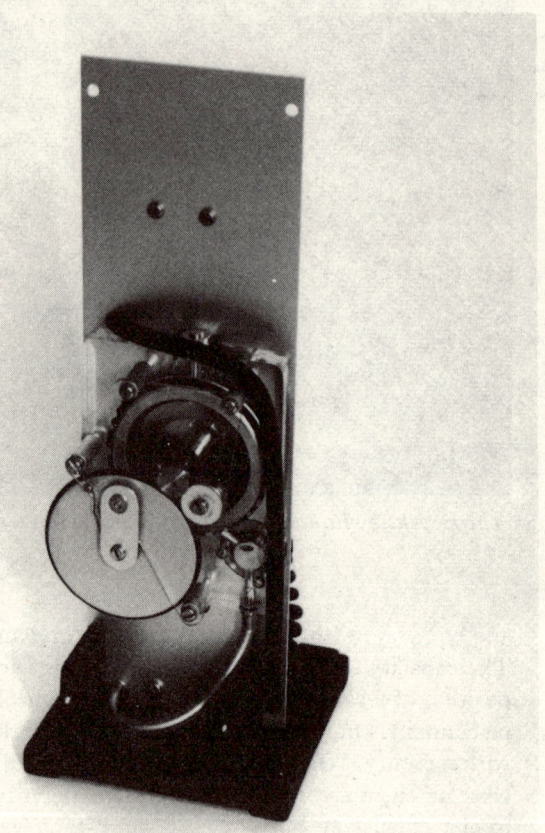

Fig. 3.6. *The Hawksley instrument showing the mechanism for varying the manometer's effective mercury content.*

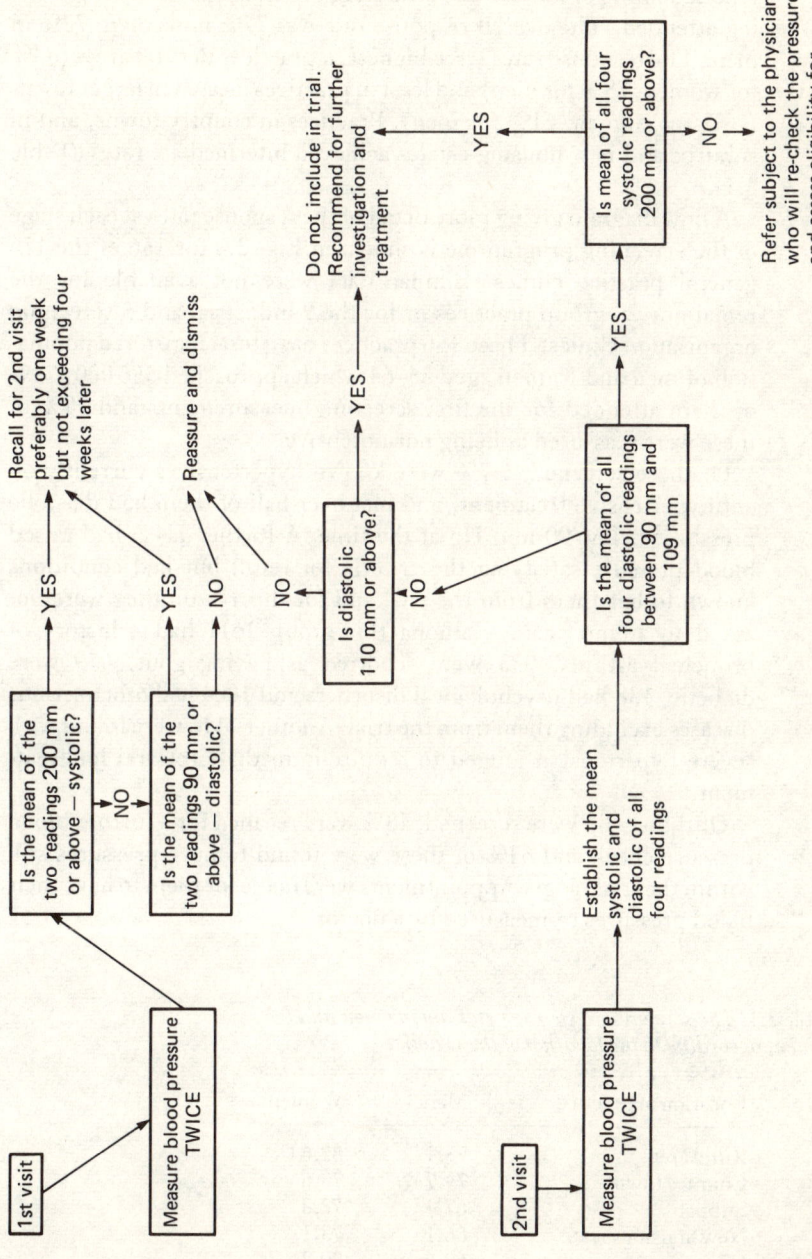

Fig. 3.7. Screening instructions.

The response rates at screening

About 500 000 of the 695 000 who were eventually invited for screening attended. The overall response rate was 77% in women, 72% in men. The response rates were highest in practices in rural areas (83% for women, 78% for men) and least in practices located in larger towns (70% for women, 61% for men). Practices in country towns, and in suburbs and new housing estates achieved intermediate rates (Table 3.1).

A flow diagram giving more detail of the response rates at each stage of the screening programme is shown in Fig. 3.8 for 156 of the 176 general practice clinics. Similar data were not available for the remaining 20 group practices or for the 9 industrial and 5 screening organisation clinics. These 156 practices has a total registered population of men and women aged 35–64 which approached 556 000; 74% of them attended for the first screening measurements and 79% of these were reassured as being normotensive.

Of those screened, 5.7% were known hypertensives currently on antihypertensive treatment, and just over half of them had diastolic pressures below 90 mm Hg at the time. A further 1.4% had raised blood pressure satisfying the criteria for recall but had conditions known to bar them from the trial and for this reason they were not asked to attend again – among this group 1611 had a history of bronchial asthma, 933 were reported as having gout, 679 were diabetic, 138 had psychological disorders and 1004 had other serious diseases excluding them from the trial. Another 1116 were found with severe hypertension judged to require immediate referral for treatment.

Of those who were screened, 13% were recalled for a further blood pressure check and 64% of these were found to have pressures still within the trial range. Appointments were made for them to have their blood pressures re-measured by a doctor.

Table 3.1. *The screening response rates among men and women, according to the location of the practice*

Location of practice	Men	Women
Rural area	78.1	82.6
Country town	74.7	78.6
Suburb	67.4	72.8
New housing estate	66.1	73.1
Conurbation	60.6	70.2
All areas	72.0	77.0

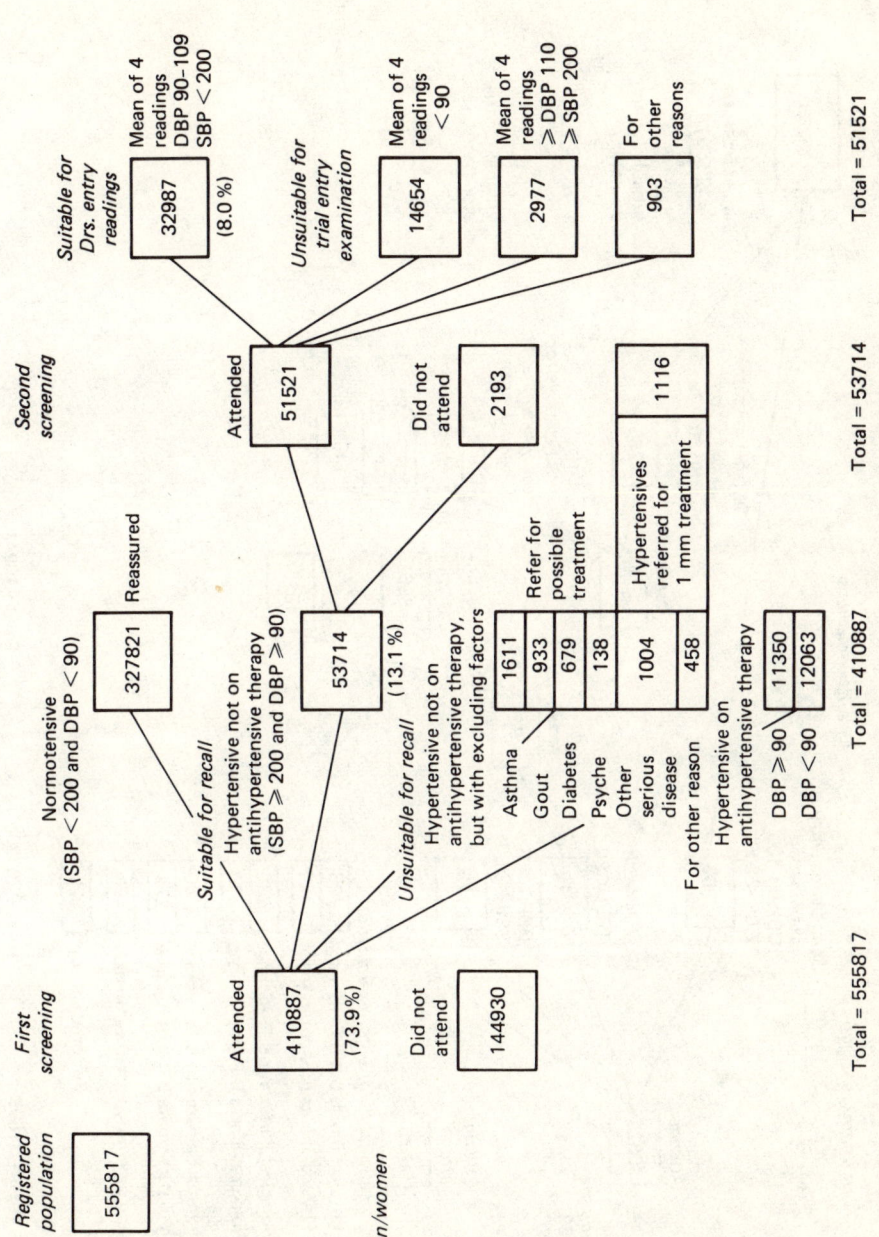

Fig. 3.8. *The response rates at screening in 156 of the 176 general practice clinics.*

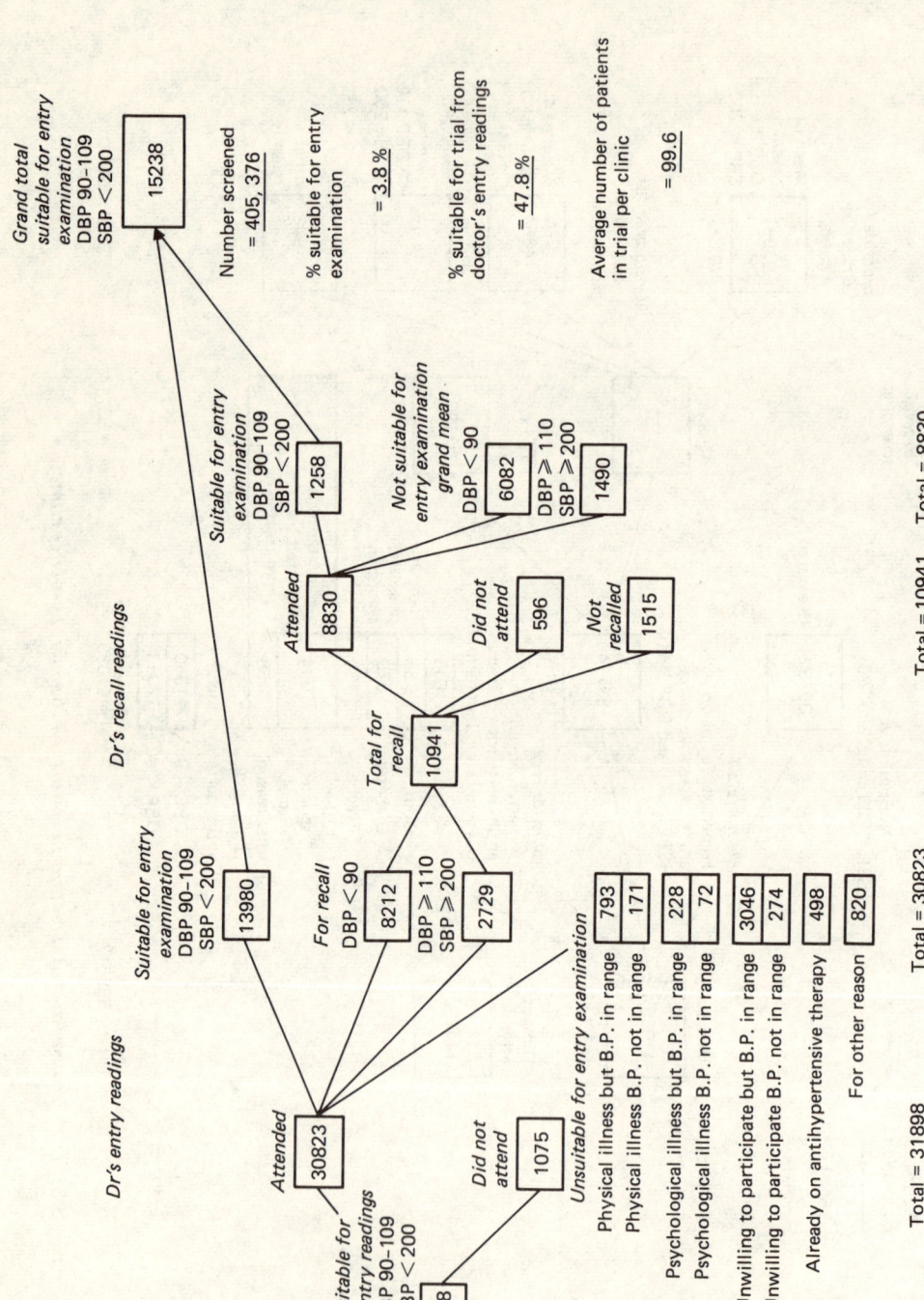

Fig. 3.9. *The response rates at the doctors' screening examinations in 153 clinics.*

A flow diagram showing the outcome in nearly 32 000 people (from 153 of these 156 clinics) who attended for the doctors' measurements is shown in Fig. 3.9. Only about 50% of those who attended retained blood pressures (after recall if necessary) within the trial range. Most of those whose pressures fell outside the criteria had shown a further drop in blood pressure.

From this group of 153 clinics, 15 238 patients were eligible for the trial entry examination, about 100 per clinic on average. This was 3.8% of those screened which was less than the 4.7% anticipated from the pilot trial experience. Eighteen general practices, already enrolled in the trial, were asked to re-screen their 35–64-year-old patients some 2 to 5 years after the initial screening. This involved another 56 000 registered people of whom only 57% responded. Another 1012 trial participants were recruited thus, and together with the previous screening brought the total number of trial entrants to 17 354.

The growth of the trial

The first person to enter the pilot trial did so in March 1973. Within 2 years of that date it was clear that the main study was feasible but the important question 'Does the trial have an adverse effect on the quality of life of its participants?' had not then been answered. For this reason, and because more data were required to allow a reliable estimate of the costs of the main study, the pilot trial was prolonged beyond its planned 2-year duration.

To maintain the impetus of the trial, recruitment was allowed to continue throughout 1975 and 1976 and funds for this were given by one of the pharmaceutical companies which provided one of the primary drug regimes, Imperial Chemical Industries Ltd. This financial help meant that the trial grew, slowly but steadily, from its pilot phase until authorisation to expand to the full-scale venture came in 1977.

The interval between the time when the Working Party had convinced itself of the feasibility of the main study (1975) and the authorisation to expand to its full-scale size (1977), was partly attributable to the pressure of other demands on the MRC's funds and this contributed to the long duration of the MRC trial. In this sort of situation once a decision has been made on feasibility no effort should be spared to increase the rate of recruitment to the maximum possible. This is when the sponsors' support is most needed if large trials are to be completed within a reasonable time. Figure 3.10 shows the number of people screened, per calendar month, from the time when mobile screening units were first used in 1976. The rate of screening increased

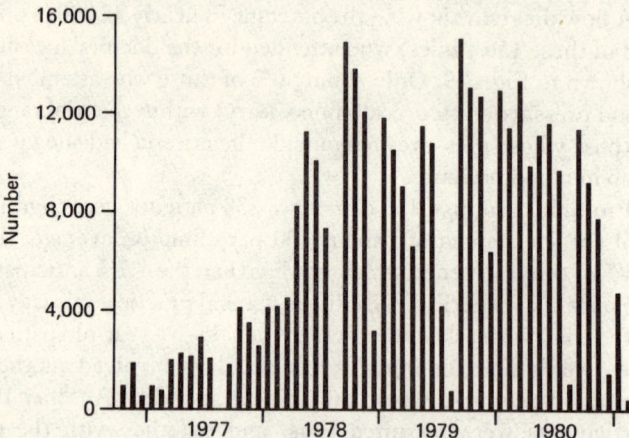

Fig. 3.10. *The numbers screened in mobile caravans per calendar month, October 1976 to February 1981.*

markedly during 1978 and in peak months over 15 000 people were being screened in this way. Figure 3.11 shows the relatively slow growth of trial entrants until early 1978 when the aim was to try to complete recruitment as fast as possible.

The role of the general practices

Drug trials in the field of hypertension conducted in general practice have been judged, frequently quite rightly, as totally inadequate. Too often general practitioners have been unfairly blamed for this. Part of the problem of drug trials sponsored by pharmaceutical companies in the past has been that the commitment required from the GP has been too small. No doubt it was often kept small deliberately so that it would not impose an excessive demand on the practitioner's time, yet these trials where each GP might enter only half a dozen patients were also so small that they required little or no assistance for the GP from the nurse or receptionist and thus, in the hurly-burly of a busy practice, could easily be forgotten or given inadequate attention.

Research-minded GPs were well aware of the deficiencies and knew that insufficient thought and planning was being given to matters such as the standardisation of measurements and methods of record keeping, the appropriate use of controls and the recording of long-term as well as short-term effects of the new drugs. Many GPs were becoming disillusioned with the sort of trials being organised by the drug firms, but the last decade has witnessed a much-needed and welcome change in the quality of some trials promoted by the pharmaceutical industry.

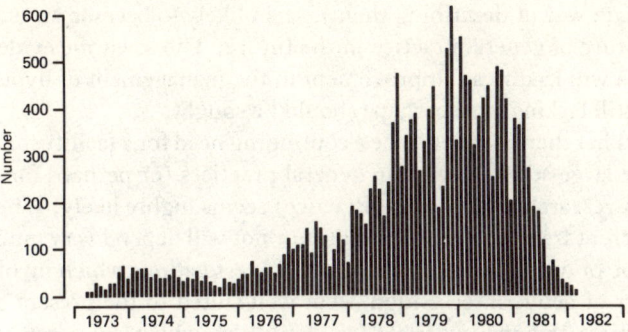

Fig. 3.11. *The numbers of new trial entrants per calendar month.*

There is no doubt that the organisational and administrative arrangements for the MRC trial were quite a success, and especially so in comparison with what had, until then, been the norm. The additional work load imposed by the trial on the average practice, once the screening phase was finished, was the regular follow-up of about 100 patients, with perhaps rather more frequent biochemical and ECG tests than would be undertaken in a non-research situation. This extra volume of work was more than most practices felt they could carry without some addition to their staff, and thus from the early days of the trial, grew the concept of appointing part-time nurses specifically for the trial work.

The success of the organisational aspects at the clinics was largely attributable to these part-time nurses and in particular the efficient team of 'training nurses'. The fact that the MRC recognised that the work would be better done if each practice realised that it was involved in a considerable commitment, and showed that it (the MRC) was willing to make the necessary funds available to ensure that adequate facilities and staff were provided, gave the trial a good reputation among most of its participating clinics. The teamwork at the periphery was matched by the keenness of the small group of 10–15 people who helped to co-ordinate the study at Northwick Park Hospital. They also were mostly women and part-timers; the majority were clerical assistants and data processors without previous experience of this kind.

The enthusiasm of the GPs and nurses undoubtedly contributed to the high compliance rates in both attendance and tablet taking. It also led to several of the practices using their 'MRC nurses' to establish clinics, under the guidance and leadership of one of the partners, first for the care of hypertensive patients who had not been in the trial and later for the continued follow-up of the trial patients after the trial had closed. These 'nurse-run' hypertension clinics (if that is an appropriate way of describing them), seem likely to become an established feature of general practice in the future. The scientific evidence that this will lead to an improvement in the management of hypertension is still lacking, and perhaps should be sought.

That there is going to be a continuing need for a facility for carrying out large-scale research in general practices (or perhaps for carrying out research into General Practice) seems highly likely. Whether the current framework is maintained or not will depend very much on the type of questions to be answered. Investigations which involve some sort of active intervention seem well suited to the present group of clinics; therapeutic trials for conditions which are common in the general population have attracted their interest and the mild hypertension trial is currently being followed by other large-scale randomised controlled trials. Within 18 months of the close of the original study, the group had grown to include 300 practices.

4 Trial participants

Those who entered the trial were clearly not a random sample of all people aged 35–64 with mild hypertension. They were initially selected by being on the lists of general practitioners who wanted to collaborate in a study of this kind and who practised in an area thought to be suitable; they were further selected in terms of their willingness to attend for screening and to enter the trial, and in having none of the characteristics listed in Table 2.1 which would bar them from entry. They were probably overrepresented by middle-class people.

This kind of selection is important when it comes to extrapolation to the population at large. It may be unjustifiable to conclude that results achieved in selected practices can be reproduced in less favourable circumstances. The trial was not designed to find a formula for the most appropriate method of detection and management of mild hypertension in the population at large, but to determine the extent to which the lowering of blood pressure would reduce morbidity and mortality. The selection factors operating in the trial were less relevant to the latter problem because randomisation to active or control treatment meant that the trial compared groups of people who differed (except in chance ways) only in the activity of the tablets prescribed.

Before entering the trial each person underwent a medical examination. Each was asked again about any previous treatment for hypertension, about angina, myocardial infarction, congestive heart failure, intermittent claudication, transient cerebral ischaemic attacks and strokes. Guidelines to encourage uniformity of diagnosis were provided in an operating manual supplied to each clinic. Other questions concerned symptoms which might be relevant to treatment with thiazides or beta-blocking drugs. Thus baseline information was obtained about, for instance, respiratory and circulatory symptoms, and a history of arthritis, which was helpful in the interpretation of possible drug-induced adverse reactions developing later. Trial entrants were also questioned about their current cigarette smoking and if women, about their use of the contraceptive pill.

Table 4.1. *The age and sex distribution of trial participants at entry*

Age group (years)	Men		Women	
	N	%	N	%
<35	32	0.4	15	0.2
35–44	2067	22.8	1251	15.1
45–54	3865	42.7	3327	40.1
55–64	3084	34.1	3713	44.7
Total	9048	100.0	8306	100.0

The medical history was followed by a physical examination and measurements of height and weight, a 12-lead resting ECG, urine and blood tests. The whole examination lasted about 40 minutes for each person; if the work was shared appropriately between doctor and nurse it required 20 minutes from each of them. Appointments were therefore made at 20-minute intervals. The doctor and nurse worked, where possible, in adjacent rooms.

Provided that no conditions which excluded them from the trial had been found during this examination, patients were allocated their randomised treatment without awaiting the results of serum bio-chemical tests or the official readings of the ECGs. A small proportion who had been entered into the study had to be excluded retrospectively as a result.

The age and sex distribution of trial participants is shown in Table 4.1. There was a greater proportion (23% compared with 15%) of men than of women below the age of 45, and a greater proportion (45% compared with 34%) of women than of men above the age 55. The overall proportions of men and women were almost equal – 52% were men.

With such large groups, and strict randomisation, the 3 treatment groups in each sex showed only small differences in any of the variables compared. Table 4.2 shows the similarity in personal charac-teristics at entry to the trial. The average age of men in the trial (50.6 years) was two years less than that of women (52.7 years). Both men and women tended to be overweight. Men of average height 173.7 cm (5 ft 7 in) weighed on average 81.4 kg (12 stone 11 lb); women of average height 160.4 cm (5 ft 3 in) weighed on average 69.9 kg (11 stone 0 lb). The younger participants in particular, and especially the younger women, included a high proportion of overweight people as is discussed later. At entry to the trial 31% of men, and 26% of women, were cigarette smokers and 18% of men and about 10% of

Table 4.2. *The comparability of the randomised treatment groups in terms of personal characteristics*

Personal characteristics	Men						Women					
	Bendrofluazide group		Propranolol group		Control group		Bendrofluazide group		Propranolol group		Control group	
Number	2238		2285		4525		2059		2118		4129	
	Mean	S.D.	Mean	S.D.	Mean	S.D.	Mean	S.D.	Mean	S.D.	Mean	S.D.
Age (y)	50.6	7.5	50.5	7.6	50.6	7.5	52.7	7.2	52.7	7.3	52.6	7.3
Height (cm)	173.7	7.1	173.5	6.9	173.7	6.9	160.3	6.3	160.5	6.1	160.4	6.4
Weight (kg)	81.5	12.1	81.4	11.8	81.2	11.8	70.2	13.0	69.8	12.9	69.8	13.0
Body mass index (wt/ht^2)	27.0	3.4	27.0	3.4	26.9	3.4	27.3	4.9	27.1	4.9	27.1	4.8
% Cigarette smokers	31.7		30.3		31.7		27.0		25.4		26.9	
% Smoking 20+ cigarettes/day	18.0		17.8		17.7		9.5		9.5		9.7	
% On contraceptive pill	—		—		—		1.2		1.0		1.1	

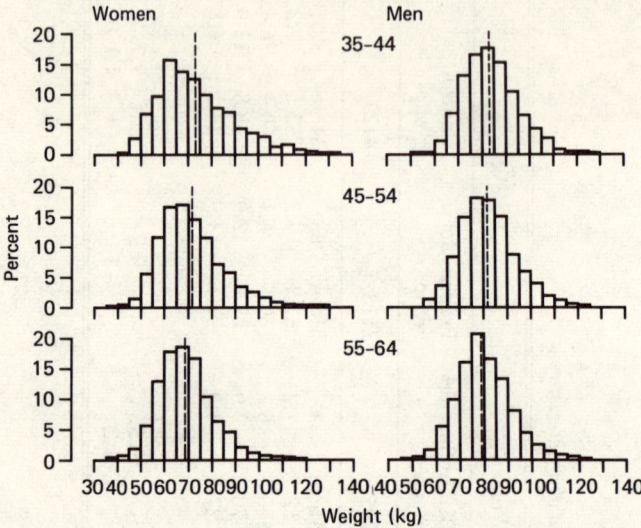

Fig. 4.1. *Distributions of body weight (kg) at entry to the trial, according to age (y) and sex.*

women were smoking 20 or more cigarettes daily. The trial entrants smoked less, and included a smaller proportion of heavy cigarette smokers, than the general population (OPCS, 1981) as would be expected of a group of relatively well-to-do subjects willing to enter a therapeutic trial.

The trial policy concerning mildly hypertensive women on the contraceptive pill was to advise them to adopt some other method of contraception. Only those who were unwilling to change, or those whose blood pressure remained raised when off the pill, were encouraged to join the trial. One per cent of women were taking the contraceptive pill at entry.

The co-ordinating centre made no attempt to influence the general advice given at clinics to trial participants with other risk factors for cardiovascular complications. The trial doctors and nurses often asked about the trial's policy on cigarette smoking, weight control, high serum cholesterol, salt intake and similar problems. They were encouraged to continue to give their usual advice on these matters but to be careful to give the same advice to treated and to control subjects, and in the final analyses it was found that the proportion of people who gave up smoking during the study was similar in the treated and untreated groups.

Cardiovascular characteristics are compared between groups in

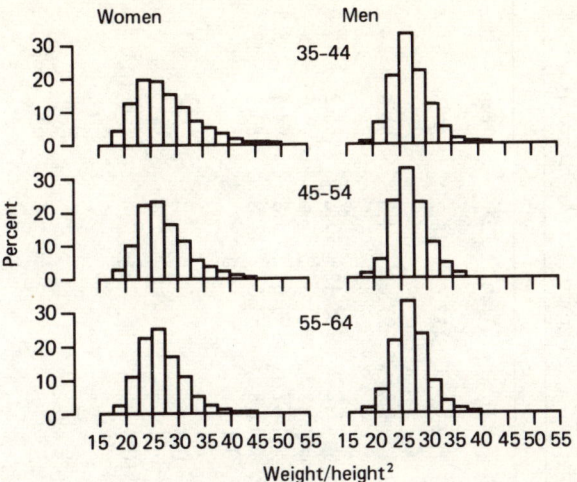

Fig. 4.2. *Distributions of Body Mass Index (kg/m²) at entry to the trial, according to age (y) and sex.*

Table 4.3. Due to the constraints on the acceptable range of diastolic pressures at screening and at entry to the trial, mean diastolic pressures were similar in the two sexes. Systolic pressures (which were not similarly constrained) were 7–8 mm Hg higher in women than in men at the entry examination. Within sexes the 3 randomised groups were closely comparable in cardiovascular characteristics.

Likewise biochemical variables showed very similar distributions between randomised groups at entry (Table 4.4). Mean values of serum cholesterol, urea, uric acid, (casual) glucose and potassium and sodium were almost identical in the 3 randomised groups in each sex; serum cholesterol levels were higher in women than in men; serum urea levels were slightly higher, and serum uric acid levels considerably higher, in men than in women. Urine biochemistry showed interesting sex differences. Proteinuria and glycosuria were both more common in the men with mild hypertension than in the women.

Distributions of body weight in trial entrants are shown, by age and sex, in Fig. 4.1. (Measurements were made with subjects clothed but without shoes or jackets.) The distributions are skewed towards higher values, particularly among women and most strikingly in the youngest age group of women. Distributions of Body Mass Index (BMI) (weight in kg divided by height², in metres) show a similar pattern (Fig. 4.2). These distributions of BMI are compared with those found in men and women of the same ages but unselected as

Table 4.3. *The comparability of the randomised treatment groups in terms of cardiovascular characteristics at entry to the trial*

Cardiovascular characteristics	Men						Women					
	Bendrofluazide group		Propranolol group		Control group		Bendrofluazide group		Propranolol group		Control group	
	Mean	S.D.	Mean	S.D.	Mean	S.D.	Mean	S.D.	Mean	S.D.	Mean	S.D.
Screening systolic pressure (mm Hg)	154.3	14.8	155.0	15.3	154.8	14.8	157.4	15.3	157.5	15.7	157.5	15.4
Screening diastolic pressure (mm Hg)	97.1	4.8	97.2	4.8	97.0	4.8	96.9	4.8	97.0	4.8	96.9	4.8
Entry systolic pressure (mm Hg)	157.6	16.3	158.2	16.3	158.2	16.4	165.3	17.2	165.4	17.2	165.2	17.0
Entry diastolic pressure (mm Hg)	98.2	5.8	98.4	5.7	98.0	5.7	98.5	5.7	98.6	5.8	98.4	5.8
Pulse rate at entry (s^{-1})	80.1	11.3	80.1	11.2	80.1	11.3	83.2	11.8	83.3	11.8	83.3	12.1
% history of previous MI	0.9		0.8		0.8		0.1		0.2		0.1	
% history of previous stroke	0.8		0.7		0.7		0.7		0.7		0.7	
% history of anti-hypertensive treatment	5.0		4.0		4.0		10.5		11.7		10.9	
% abnormal Q/QS complexes (Minnesota code 1_1 & 1_2)	1.0		1.2		1.5		1.7		1.7		1.4	
% abnormal S-T & T changes (Minnesota code $4_{1-3}5_{1-2}$)	1.3		1.0		1.1		2.1		1.3		1.7	

Table 4.4. *The comparability of the randomised treatment groups in terms of biochemical characteristics at entry to the trial*

Biochemical characteristics	Men						Women					
	Bendrofluazide group		Propranolol group		Control group		Bendrofluazide group		Propranolol group		Control group	
	Mean	S.D.	Mean	S.D.	Mean	S.D.	Mean	S.D.	Mean	S.D.	Mean	S.D.
Serum cholesterol (mmol/l)	6.3	1.1	6.3	1.0	6.3	1.0	6.7	1.2	6.7	1.2	6.7	1.2
Serum urea (mmol/l)	5.4	1.2	5.4	1.2	5.4	1.2	5.2	1.2	5.1	1.2	5.2	1.2
Serum urate (μmol/l)	381.9	69.7	373.9	68.6	373.4	66.0	296.9	65.8	293.3	61.6	293.1	61.1
Serum glucose (mmol/l)	5.5	1.1	5.5	1.1	5.4	1.0	5.4	0.9	5.4	1.0	5.4	0.9
Serum potassium (mmol/l)	4.1	0.4	4.1	0.4	4.2	0.4	4.1	0.4	4.1	0.4	4.1	0.4
Serum sodium (mmol/l)	147.7	2.2	141.6	2.3	141.7	2.2	141.6	2.3	141.8	2.1	141.7	3.1
% Proteinuria												
Trace	4.8		4.6		4.6		3.2		3.1		3.7	
Definite	0.7		0.5		0.9		0.3		0.8		0.4	
% Glycosuria												
Trace	0.3		0.4		0.5		0.0		0.1		0.2	
Definite	0.1		0.1		0.1		0.0		0.0		0.0	

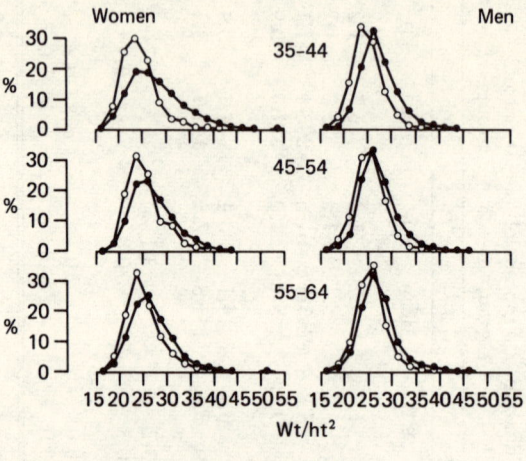

Fig. 4.3. *A comparison of the distributions of Body Mass Index (kg/m²) in the trial population and in a sample of the general population unselected by blood pressure – data from the Northwick Park Heart Study.*

regards blood pressure, in Fig. 4.3. The comparative population is that of the Northwick Park Heart Study (Meade *et al.*, 1980), a prospective study of representative men and women in the general population of N.W. London.

The blood pressure criteria of the trial clearly resulted in the selection into it of overweight people of both sexes, as would be expected, but the picture differs between the sexes. In men the distributions of body build are similar in the two populations, but shifted towards higher values in the hypertensive men; in women, and particularly in young women, the distribution is not only shifted towards higher values in the hypertensive subjects but is also markedly more skewed.

The relationship between body weight and blood pressure, as is discussed later, is closer in women than it is in men. This is true in the trial data and accords with the findings of epidemiological studies of the general population (Miall, Bell and Lovell, 1968). It is also greater in younger than in older subjects. These relationships must mean that younger women with blood pressures at a level making them eligible for the trial would tend to be overweight.

This type of selection disturbs the usual relationships between variables and not only complicates the analysis of longitudinal data, as will be mentioned in Chapter 5, but also makes a trial control group, influenced as it also is by trial entry and withdrawal criteria, an inappropriate population for a study of the natural history of untreated mild hypertension.

The trial was not intended to be used as an epidemiological study of factors influencing mild hypertension and from the outset we determined not to collect a lot of information which might never be analysed. Both the information obtained by questioning participants and the number of biochemical investigations carried out were restricted to what was considered essential. With hindsight we realised that some of the limitations were unwise. For example, no information was sought about the social or educational status of the participants and the data on employment included only brief details of the nature and place of work and were intended mainly to assist with follow-up. It might have been useful to see which social factors, if any, influenced lapse rates, compliance with therapy and good blood pressure control. Nothing was asked about alcohol intake, for example, and likewise no information was collected on family history of arterial disease and though such information is often unreliable and difficult to interpret, it might have had value in defining groups at particularly increased risk.

Some participants in the trial finished their stints before the trial as a whole was ready to be stopped. This gave a valuable opportunity to see to what extent the benefits of long-term antihypertensive treatment persisted after treatment was withdrawn. Those who were willing to take part in this further study were re-randomised (at their sixth anniversary of entry to the trial), to groups which either continued or discontinued taking their tablets whether these were active drugs or placebo. This so-called 'Phase II study' showed the rates at which pressures returned towards untreated levels in the different groups, and the rates of return to normal values of the biochemical abnormalities induced by the drugs. There was no evidence of any sizeable group whose baroreceptors had been permanently reset to a clinically important extent. The antihypertensive effects had almost disappeared within a year of stopping treatment, as a result of a general shift of the distribution of pressures towards a higher level; the biochemical abnormalities were largely resolved within two years of withdrawal (MRC Working Party, 1986*b*).

5 Treatment groups and the course of blood pressure

In Britain the two groups of drugs most frequently used for controlling mild hypertension at the start of the trial (and also 12 years later when it finished) were the thiazide diuretics and the beta-adrenergic blocking agents. But a lively, interesting and at times heated discussion took place about the manner in which these two drugs should be used in the trial. Some advocated a combined beta-blocker/thiazide regime. Had that view prevailed the trial would have generated data which would, in effect, have been more relevant to what had become current practice by the time the trial ended. This could not have been predicted. The other view was that the trial would provide more valuable data by using the two regimes separately. The comparison of two drugs of different classes would give an opportunity to separate the benefits attributable to the reduction in blood pressure *per se* from those attributable to other effects of the drugs. In fact the latter view prevailed and allowed comparisons of the effects of the separate regimes which became such an interesting feature of the trial results. But it is still debatable whether the right decision was made and it would take another similar trial to answer that question. Bendrofluazide was the thiazide selected for the trial, being very widely used with no known serious irreversible adverse reactions, and cheap; for similar reasons, propranolol was the beta-blocker chosen. Both drugs had been on the market for more than 10 years.

Although the trial was designed to determine the effects of blood pressure reduction on cardiovascular complications rather than to compare the efficacy of two types of antihypertensive drugs with very different modes of action, it seemed sensible to plan the study in such a way as to provide as much useful information as possible about their separate values. One particular reason for wanting to be able to look at the effects of the drugs separately was that the MRC trial was the first real opportunity to see whether the beta-blockers would be useful in the primary prevention of the coronary complications of hypertension.

As it turned out, by the time the trial finished it had provided grounds for believing that sub-groups of the population reacted differently to the two treatments and it was a relief to be able to look at the data without the effects of one drug being seriously contaminated by those of the other. So despite the fact that drugs of these two types were commonly used in general practice to supplement one another when blood pressure proved hard to control, this was against protocol in the trial and doctors were asked to contact the co-ordinating centre before doing so. Methyl dopa (and originally, though much less in later years, guanethidine) were used as supplementary drugs.

Bendrofluazide, with a comparatively flat dose/response curve, was to be given in a fixed dose 5 mg b.d. – a dose which now and with hindsight seems high but at that time was believed would be more effective than a smaller one. It was also believed that this dose would correspond in its blood pressure lowering properties with what was thought likely to be the usual dose of propranolol employed, 40 mg b.d. The possible importance of thiazide dose in relation to the development of adverse reactions was not then fully understood.

For propranolol, the dose was not fixed. All participants started with a test dose, and the majority were subsequently found to be well controlled on 40 mg b.d. If necessary, however, and in the absence of marked bradycardia, the clinic nurses were encouraged to increase the dose stepwise to 120 mg b.d., or up to 160 mg b.d. exceptionally, before considering the addition of supplementary methyl dopa or guanethidine.

The aim of therapy for patients on active treatment was to control the diastolic pressure below 90 mm Hg. A patient showing a limited response at 12 weeks after entering the trial (i.e. pressure lower than at entry but still above 95 mm Hg) could continue on the primary drug regime and was seen at monthly intervals with the possibility of then having a supplementary drug added. A patient showing no response by 8 weeks was to be started on supplementary therapy at that stage.

Blood pressure response to treatment

Figures 5.1 and 5.2 show the proportion of men and women whose diastolic pressures were at target levels (below 90 mm Hg) at each annual examination. On each occasion about 40% of control men, and a slightly higher proportion of control women, had diastolic pressures at target – i.e. below the range which allowed them into the trial. The proportion was similar in each age group. Though the proportion remained fairly constant throughout the trial, the individuals comprising the group differed from one occasion to the next. The phenomenon was a manifestation of the variability of arterial pressure.

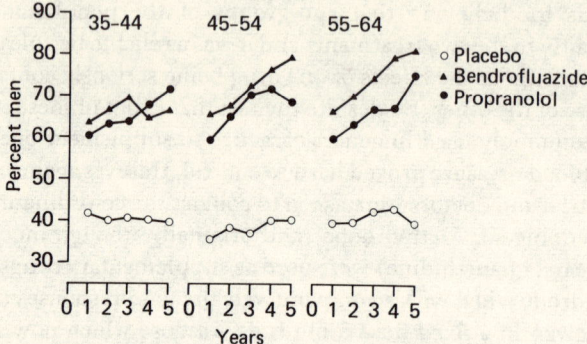

Fig. 5.1. *The proportions of men with diastolic pressures at target, according to randomised treatment regime, age and time in the trial.*

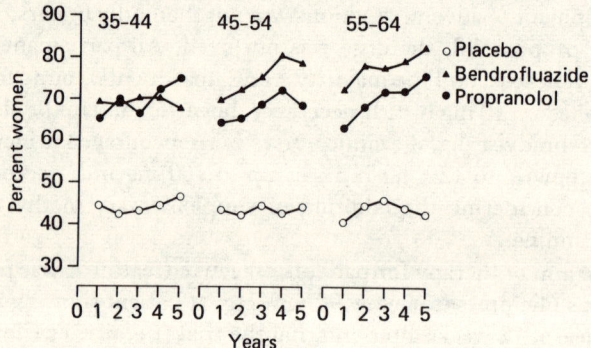

Fig. 5.2. *As for Fig. 5.1, but for women.*

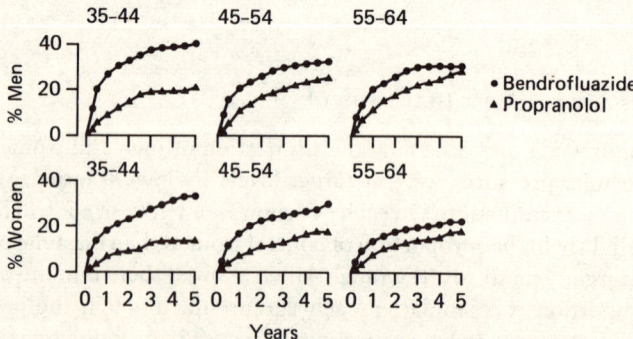

Fig. 5.3. *Cumulative percentages of men and women requiring supplementary therapy according to randomised treatment regime, age (y) and time in the trial.*

Among those on active treatment, and in both sexes and in each age group, the proportion at target pressure increased during the course of the trial in both treatment groups. The proportion at target pressure increased with age at entry among those taking bendrofluazide but was independent of age in the propranolol group; as a result, there was a consistently higher proportion of 45–54- and 55–64-year-olds in the thiazide group at target than in those receiving the beta-blocker.

The trial seemed to be supporting earlier evidence that thiazides controlled blood pressure more effectively in older people than beta-blockers. Comparison of the two treatment regimes in the trial is complicated by the use of supplementary drugs which were introduced to a greater extent, and earlier, in thiazide takers than in the beta-blocker group. Figure 5.3 shows the proportion of men and women in the 3 age groups, according to their randomised treatment regime, who required supplementary therapy. Although the proportions were consistently higher in the fixed dose bendrofluazide group than in the propranolol group where the dose was titrated before introducing a supplement, the need for supplementary drugs in the thiazide takers was greatest in the younger and least in the older age groups of both sexes, whereas no comparable trend was apparent in those taking the beta-blocker.

Mean systolic and diastolic pressures at entry to the trial, 3 months after entry, and thereafter at annual examinations, are shown in Figs. 5.4 and 5.5. After the initial fall in pressure which occurred in both treated and control subjects, mean systolic pressure in control subjects tended to rise throughout the trial, but never reached entry levels; in those actively treated it remained constant or tended to fall. Mean diastolic pressure remained about constant in control subjects but tended to fall to lower values among the treated.

The differences in pressures between treated and control subjects, resulting from these trends are summarised in Table 5.1. It is clear that the separation in pressure between treated and controls was greater in older than in younger subjects, in those on bendrofluazide than in those on propranolol and, particularly in the older age groups, increased with time in the trial. The only notable sex difference in response is seen in 35–44-year olds, where the pressure differences between treated and controls were greater in women than in men.

Interpretation of these blood pressure trends in the different groups requires caution. Figures 5.4 and 5.5 show the mean pressures according to treatment groups as randomised. With the passage of time more and more people on active tablets had been started on supplementary drugs, and the use of supplements differed according to primary drug regime, differed in the two sexes and, in the case of

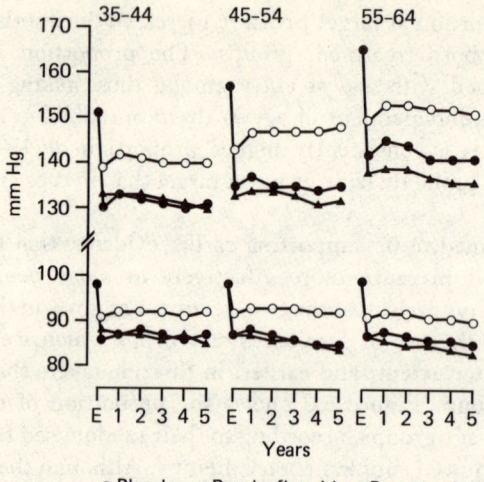

Fig. 5.4. *Mean systolic and diastolic pressures in men according to randomised treatment regime, age (y) and time in the trial.*

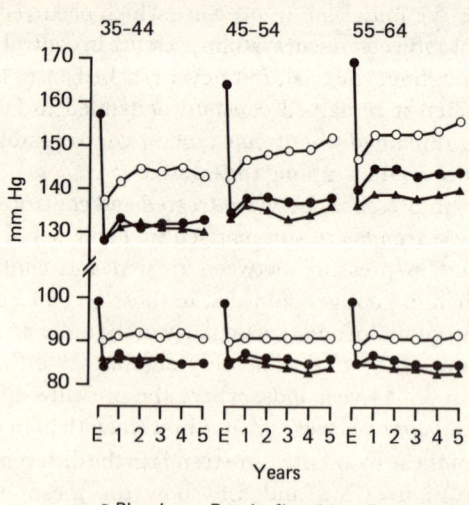

Fig. 5.5. *As for Fig. 5.4, but for women.*

Table 5.1. Net differences in systolic and diastolic pressures (mm Hg) between treated and control subjects,[a] according to age, sex and time in the trial

	Year	35–44		45–54		55–64	
		Bendrofluazide	Propranolol	Bendrofluazide	Propranolol	Bendrofluazide	Propranolol
Systolic							
Men	1	8.7	8.7	11.8	9.8	13.8	8.3
	2	8.5	9.0	12.9	11.2	14.0	9.2
	3	7.8	8.5	14.1	12.8	15.3	12.2
	4	8.0	9.1	16.3	14.4	14.9	11.3
	5	7.3	7.2	17.3	13.0	14.3	12.0
Women	1	11.8	9.0	11.6	9.5	14.1	7.8
	2	12.7	12.7	12.1	10.2	15.1	8.9
	3	12.8	9.4	15.1	11.8	15.3	10.0
	4	17.3	10.8	15.6	12.2	15.3	12.0
	5	14.5	8.7	15.3	12.3	16.4	15.8
Diastolic							
Men	1	4.0	4.9	6.2	5.4	6.2	4.6
	2	4.5	4.8	6.6	5.9	7.1	4.9
	3	4.6	5.1	7.2	6.8	7.3	5.4
	4	4.3	5.7	7.4	7.2	8.7	5.9
	5	5.1	5.7	9.2	7.6	8.4	5.6
Women	1	5.1	4.5	5.0	4.5	6.9	4.6
	2	5.6	7.0	5.8	4.8	7.2	5.0
	3	6.5	6.5	6.8	6.1	7.4	5.4
	4	6.9	7.9	7.3	6.9	9.1	6.4
	5	5.8	6.7	7.2	6.6	9.5	8.0

[a] Change in pressure in treated minus change in pressure in controls, since entry.

bendrofluazide, differed in the 3 age groups. It is also possible that methyl dopa (the most commonly used supplement) is more effective when used with a thiazide than when used with a beta-blocker. Likewise an increasing number of control subjects had to be transferred to active therapy during the trial, as discussed in Chapter 6; the inclusion of their blood pressure data in Figures 5.4 and 5.5 must mean that the rise in pressure of untreated controls would have been greater.

The drop in blood pressure following entry to the trial

The sharp drop in pressure during the first 3 months in the trial occurred even among placebo-treated control subjects and was present in every age and sex group. Some drop in pressure following entry was anticipated, but the size of the fall was greater than expected and it continued for longer than seemed likely. Most of it occurred between the entry medical examination and the first follow-up visit two weeks later, but the fall was sustained in a more gradual form for the next 10 weeks. To some extent the size of the drop in pressure shown in Figs. 5.4 and 5.5 is exaggerated by the pressor effect of the entry examination itself. Pressures were higher then, when taken by doctors, than they had been at the screening, particularly among women (Table 5.2).

The possibility that the fall in pressure among controls was a true placebo effect of taking tablets was investigated in a sub-study in which about 300 people in the control group were assigned randomly to attend for observations only, taking no tablets. There was no difference between the course of blood pressure in this group and in the placebo tablet takers (illustrated for women in Fig. 5.6), and this 'observation only' group, which formed part of the control group, will not be further described here. The fall in pressure was clearly related to factors other than tablet-taking, of which regression towards the

Table 5.2. *Mean systolic and diastolic pressures at screening and at entry examination in men and women*

		Systolic (mm Hg)	Diastolic (mm Hg)
Men:	Screening	155	97
	Entry	158	98
Women:	Screening	157	97
	Entry	165	99

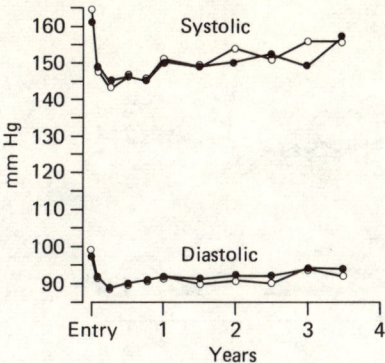

Fig. 5.6. *Mean systolic and diastolic pressures of two groups of control women – a placebo group (○) and an observation group (●).*

mean and habituation to clinic procedures were likely to be the most significant. As most of the change occurred within the first two weeks regression towards the mean was presumably the more important.

The value of methyl dopa as a supplementary drug

After 5 years in the trial 34% of men and 24% of women on bendrofluazide had been started on supplementary therapy. In the propranolol group the proportions were 25% of men and 18% of women. The use of supplementary therapy was significantly lower in women than in men. Target pressure was achieved within 6 to 12 months of requiring supplementary methyl dopa by 55% to 60% of subjects and in 75% to 80% of those on supplementary therapy, methyl dopa was continued for at least 6 to 12 months to maintain better blood pressure control.

Factors influencing blood pressure levels

An unexpected finding when the mean blood pressure levels were plotted at 6-monthly intervals was that the values obtained at the annual examinations were consistently higher than those at the 6-monthly intermediate visits (Figs. 5.7 and 5.8). It was thought at first that the additional stress associated with the annual visit which included a physical examination, ECG, blood test, and blood pressure measurements made by doctors instead of nurses, was enough to account for the findings.

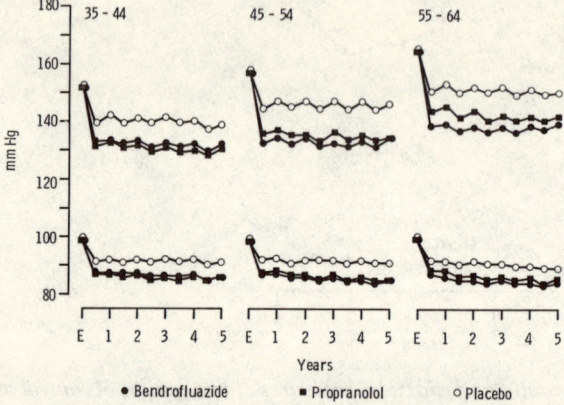

Fig. 5.7. *Mean systolic and diastolic pressures in men, recorded at 6-month intervals, according to randomised treatment regime, age (y) and time in the trial.*

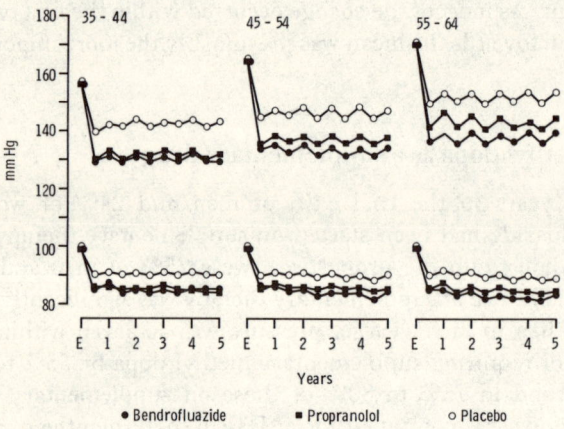

Fig. 5.8. *As for Fig. 5.7, but for women.*

Table 5.3. *The effects on systolic and diastolic (V) pressure of a 20°C difference in maximum environmental air temperature in persons aged 35 and 65, according to their body build*

	Systolic difference (mm Hg)	Diastolic difference (mm Hg)
Aged 35: Thin	2.3	2.4
Obese	1.9	1.9
Aged 65: Thin	6.7	3.5
Obese	6.2	3.1

Later in the course of the trial it became clear that there was an additional and more interesting explanation. Seasonal variation in blood pressure, with higher values in the winter than in the summer had previously been reported (Rose, 1961; Heller, Rose, Tunstall Pedoe and Christie, 1978; Hata, Ogihara, Maruyama *et al.*, 1982) but had never attracted much medical attention. The trial data provided a good opportunity to investigate seasonal variation in mean values of systolic and diastolic pressure in the two sexes. Measurements made at annual and intermediate follow-up visits were first analysed separately. Mean values were calculated according to the month in which the readings had been made. They showed not only the higher levels at the annual visits but seasonal variation superimposed upon both sets of measurements (Fig. 5.9). More of the trial participants had entered the study in the winter months than in the summer; there were therefore two reasons for the increased values at the annual visits – first, an increment attributable to the slight anxiety associated with a full medical examination and second, a greater proportion of winter measurements.

After correcting for the differences accounted for by the pressor effect of annual examinations, the results shown in Fig. 5.10 were obtained; these showed the size of the seasonal variation in the two sexes and suggested that the effect was greater in older than in younger subjects.

The relationship between blood pressure levels and meteorological data was then examined using information provided by the Meteorological Office. It was possible in this way to examine how a person's blood pressure deviated from his or her average pressure according to the environmental temperature and rainfall which had been recorded on the same day. In every age group of both sexes there was a highly significant negative correlation between either maximum or minimum daily temperature and systolic or diastolic pressure – the lower the temperature the higher the pressure. After allowing for temperature there was no residual association with rainfall. The effects of age, sex, mean blood pressure level, and body mass index on this relationship with environmental temperature were also investigated. Significant interactions were found only with age and with body mass index – the older the person, and the less protected from the cold by subcutaneous fat, the greater the change in blood pressure associated with a given change in temperature. The size of the effect is shown in Table 5.3. For a thin 65-year-old of either sex a 20°C difference in maximum air temperature would be associated with a 6.7 mm Hg change in systolic, or a 3.5 mm Hg change in diastolic, pressure (Brennan, Greenberg, Miall and Thompson, 1982).

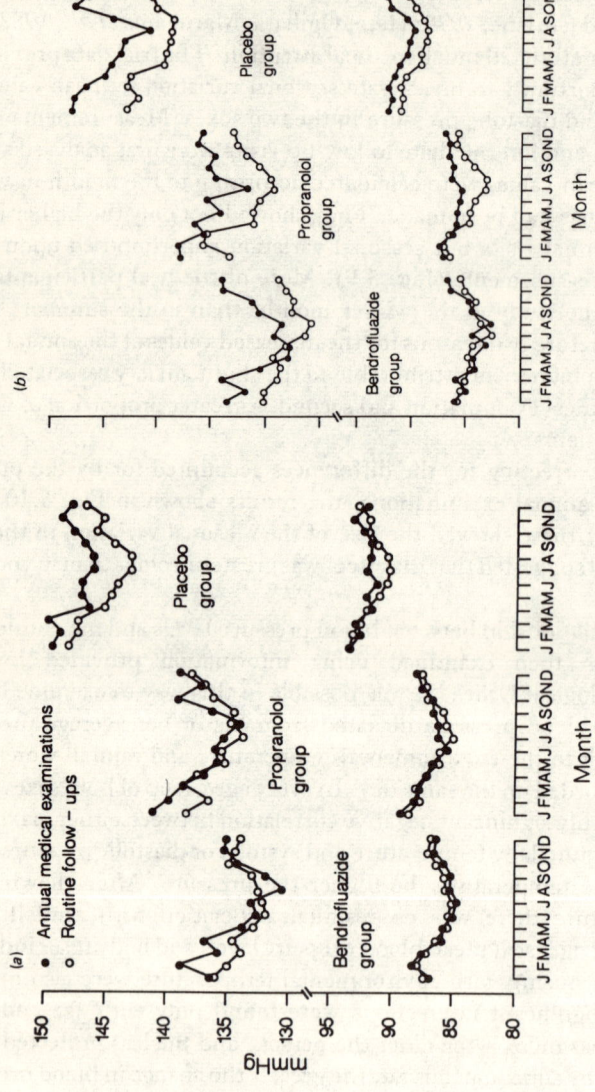

Fig. 5.9a. Mean systolic and diastolic pressures in men, recorded at annual and routine follow-up visits, according to the month of blood pressure measurement and randomised treatment regime.

Fig. 5.9b. As for Fig. 5.9a, but for women.

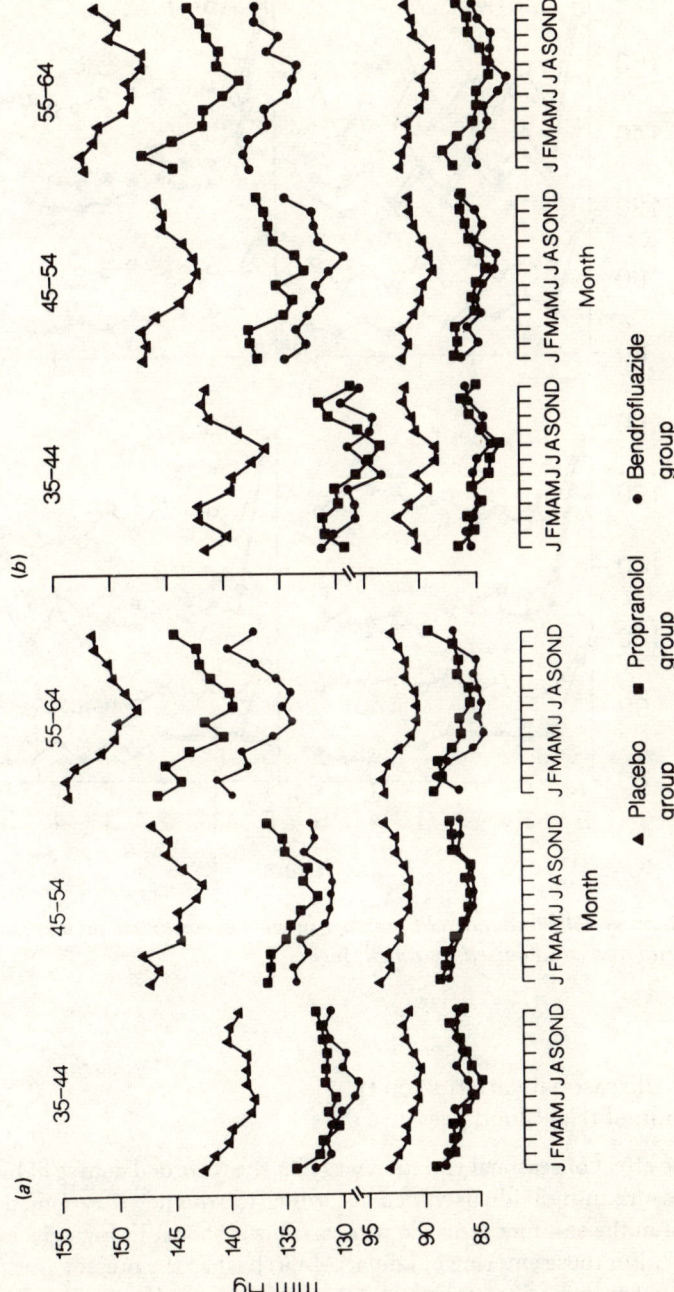

Fig. 5.10a. *Seasonal trends in systolic and diastolic pressures in men according to randomised treatment regime and age.*

Fig. 5.10b. *As for Fig. 5.10a, but for women.*

▲ Placebo group   ■ Propranolol group   ● Bendrofluazide group

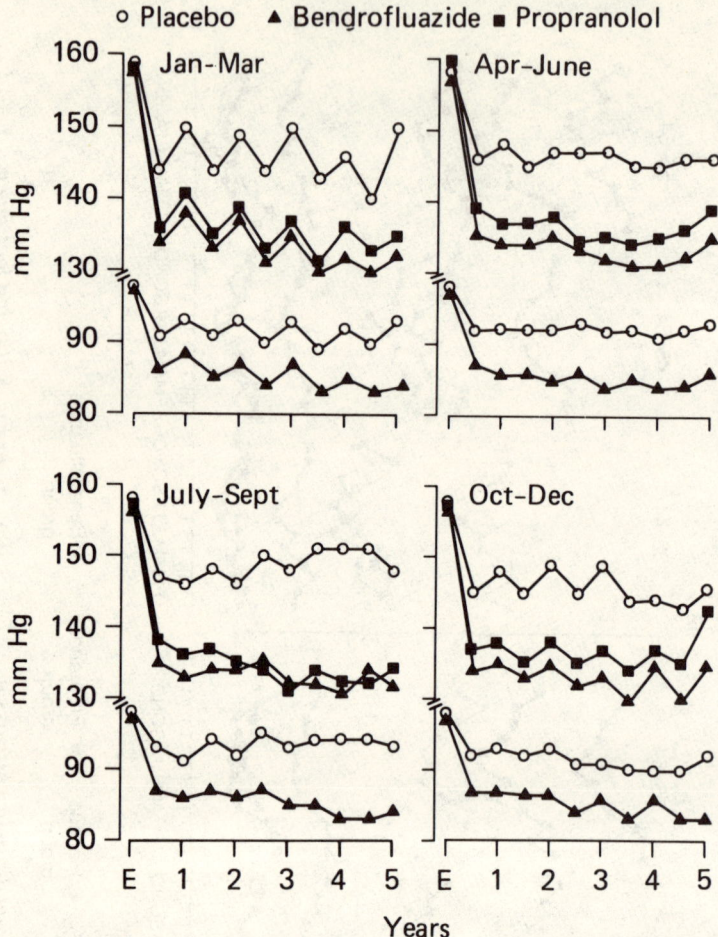

Fig. 5.11. *Mean systolic and diastolic pressure in men, according to their season of entry to the trial and randomised treatment regime.*

The effects of seasonal variation on the interpretation of trial blood pressure data

One effect of seasonal variation was that the recorded course of blood pressure in individuals varied according to whether they joined the trial in the summer or in the winter. This is shown in Figs. 5.11 and 5.12. For those entering in January–March when the pressor effects of annual examinations augmented those of cold weather, and to a lesser extent for those joining in October–December, mean pressures as

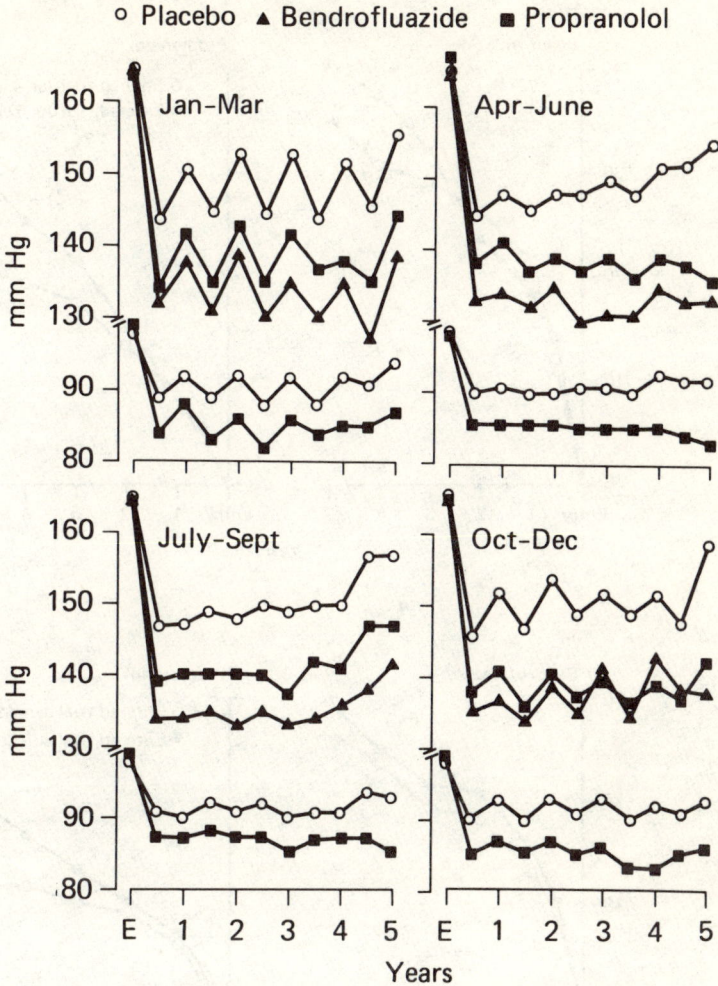

○ Placebo ▲ Bendrofluazide ■ Propranolol

Fig. 5.12. *As for Fig. 5.11, but for women.*

recorded at 6-month intervals appeared to follow a markedly zig-zag course. For those entering in April–June the curves were smoother, and for those joining the trial during July–September the pressor effects of annual visits were more than counterbalanced by the troughs in blood pressure associated with warm weather.

Another possible effect of seasonal variation would be that those whose blood pressures met trial criteria in the summer, when their blood pressures would have been below their average levels, would be somewhat more severely hypertensive than those meeting trial criteria

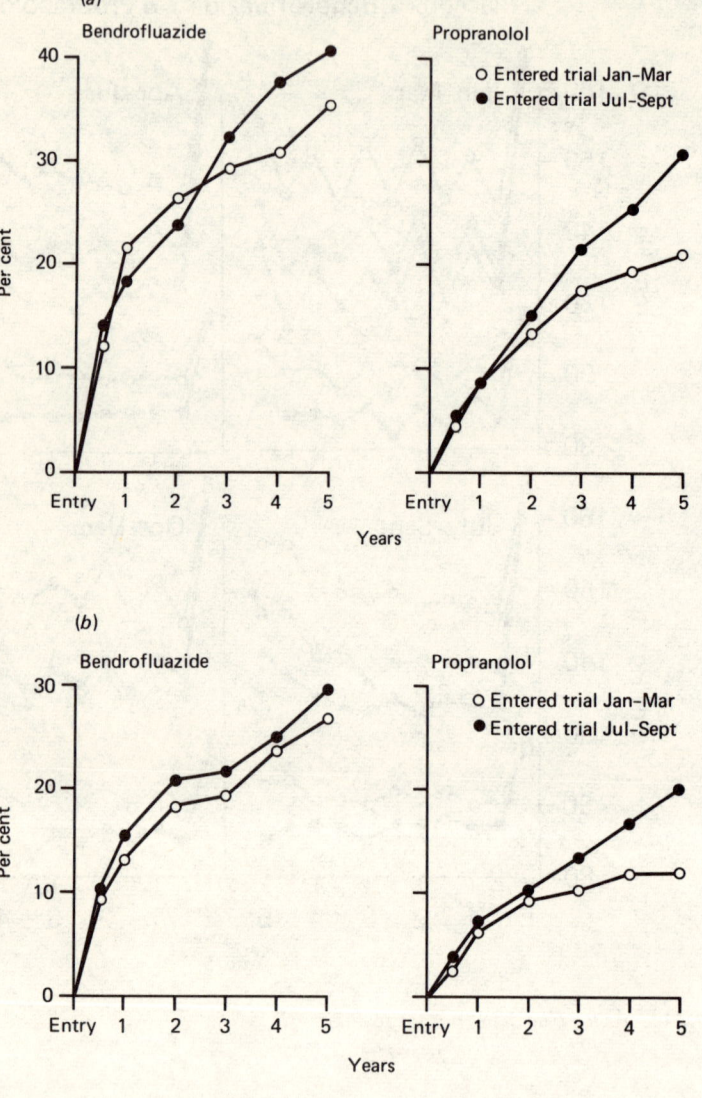

Fig. 5.13. *Cumulative percentages of men (a) and women (b) requiring supplementary drugs, according to their season of entry to the trial and randomised treatment regime.*

on their above-average winter levels. There was some evidence that this was so; a higher proportion of summer entrants than of winter entrants required supplementary drug therapy during the course of the study (Fig. 5.13).

The influence of personal factors
on blood pressure levels

Multiple linear regression analyses of factors influencing blood pressure levels at entry to the trial were carried out for each age and sex group and for systolic and diastolic pressure separately. The variables included were age, height, weight, pulse rate, cigarette smoking and certain serum biochemical characteristics.

There were 3 major problems in the interpretation of the results. First, as was to be expected in a study based on these large numbers, some correlations were statistically significant but of doubtful biological importance. These less-interesting relationships have been omitted from this discussion. Second, the population which met the trial entry requirements differed from the general population from which it was drawn in many ways other than in their blood pressures, such as their different distributions of body weight. Third, the constraints on diastolic pressure at entry, and the use of a specified level of diastolic pressure as the goal of treatment, inevitably distorted the relationships between diastolic pressure and the variables studied; because of the design of the study, systolic pressure was affected to a much smaller extent by the same problem. These factors interfere with the use of the trial data for a study of the influence of personal factors on blood pressure levels; with this caveat in mind, however, it is worth examining the results of these analyses.

In both sexes, and in all 3 treatment groups, age was by far the most important variable affecting the level of systolic pressure in cross-sectional analysis at entry (Table 5.4). Partly for the reasons given above, age had much less effect on diastolic pressure. Women, at entry to the trial and at later stages, had higher systolic pressures than did

Table 5.4. *The influence of various personal factors on blood pressure levels at entry to the trial*

Personal factors	Systolic pressure regression coefficient (mm Hg on factor)		Diastolic pressure regression coefficient (mm Hg on factor)	
	Men	Women	Men	Women
Age (10 years)	7.5***	6.6***	0.3***	0.2*
Height (10 cm)	N.S.	0.9**	0.2*	N.S.
Weight (10 kg)	−0.3*	N.S.	0.2**	0.1*
Pulse rate (10 beats/min)	1.0***	1.3***	0.2***	0.2**
Smoking/non-smoking	1.1***	N.S.	N.S.	N.S.

*** $P < 0.001$ ** $P < 0.01$ * $P < 0.05$; NS, not significant.

men; again this did not apply to diastolic pressures because of the entry constraints.

Somewhat surprisingly, an inverse relationship was found between body weight and systolic pressure – the greater the weight the lower the pressure; when age was taken into account the negative relationship diminished in men and became non-significant in women. This unusual inverse relationship between blood pressure and body weight was explained by the high proportion of young obese people – especially among women. The pressures of these young women were below the average for all women in the trial but their weights were above average.

Pulse rates were consistently and positively related to the levels of both systolic and diastolic pressure in the entry data in both sexes and this relationship was maintained in cross-sectional analyses of data collected subsequently, except in the propranolol group in which the effect of the drug in causing bradycardia obscured the underlying relationship.

In epidemiological surveys of the general population the blood pressures of smokers have been found to be lower than those of non-smokers, a finding usually attributed to the marked difference in weight between smokers and non-smokers.

In the trial the findings were different. As shown in Tables 10.1 and 10.2 in both sexes the systolic and diastolic pressures of smokers, at entry to the trial, were closely similar to those for non-smokers; and smokers weighed on average 2–3 kg less than non-smokers. After correcting for weight, the pressures of cigarette smokers were marginally higher than those of non-smokers.

This difference between the findings in the trial and the findings reported from observational studies seemed to be best explained as another manifestation of the distorting effects of the constraints on the range of blood pressures at entry. Any subdivision of the trial population, as for example by age, sex, weight, or smoking habits, would of necessity produce groups of people whose blood pressures had been limited by the narrow range of diastolic pressures acceptable for the trial. (This in turn would also indirectly constrain the systolic range.) Thus the trial data would be bound to show altered relationships between any variables and entry blood pressure levels from those that would be seen in the general population. For this reason it did not seem likely to be rewarding to pursue this type of investigation further.

To a lesser extent the longitudinal data derived from the follow-up will be distorted similarly by the same constraints which influence the analyses of the entry data. The relationships between changes in body weight and changes in blood pressure were as would be predicted,

Table 5.5. *The influence of various personal factors on blood pressure changes from entry to one year in controls*

Personal factors	Systolic pressure (mm Hg) Regression coefficient		Diastolic pressure (mm Hg) Regression coefficient	
	Men	Women	Men	Women
Age (10 years)	−1.5***	−1.7***	N.S.	N.S.
Weight (10 kg)	0.7**	0.7**	N.S.	N.S.
Weight change (10 kg)	4.5***	4.0***	2.5***	2.2***
Mean systolic pressure (10 mm Hg)	0.7***	0.9***	—	—
Mean diastolic pressure (10 mm Hg)	—	—	6.9***	6.9***

*** $P < 0.001$ ** $P < 0.01$

with gain in weight (on average) always being associated with gain in pressure. Indeed of the variables examined, change in weight usually made the greatest contribution to the extent of the change in pressure occurring during a given time (Table 5.5). The relationship between change of weight and change of pressure was statistically significant in all groups except among women treated with propranolol, where again the effect of the drug in causing an increase in weight might obscure the underlying relationships between weight and pressure.

Changes in pulse rate were not significantly related to changes in blood pressure in the analyses of longitudinal data.

Among control subjects the difference in pressure between smokers and non-smokers persisted, tending to increase slightly after entry. In the bendrofluazide-treated group the difference was rarely significant after entry. However in the propranolol-treated group the differences tended to increase after entry, particularly in women. Blood pressures on average were less well controlled by propranolol in smokers than in non-smokers.

Whatever the explanation of these small differences in the effects of the two drugs on the blood pressures of smokers and non-smokers, there is reason to believe that there is an interaction between smoking and the effects of the drugs on cardiovascular complications, and this is described in Chapter 10.

6 Withdrawals from randomised treatment

The principal reasons for withdrawal from the treatment to which participants were randomly allocated at entry fell into two groups. Those taking active tablets were withdrawn largely due to the development of a suspected adverse drug reaction and were usually then transferred to the alternative regime. Those taking the placebo tablets were withdrawn largely on the development of a level of blood pressure such that their continued management on inactive tablets became unethical; they were then usually transferred to treatment with the corresponding active regime. Other reasons for withdrawal from randomised treatment included the development of complications requiring active therapy. All patients whose treatment was changed were asked to continue to attend for all the routine follow-up examinations.

The trial provided interesting information on drug adverse reactions. It was possible not only to compare the incidence of adverse reactions in people taking either bendrofluazide or propranolol with the incidence of similar complaints in people taking placebo tablets, and to compare the two active drugs with one another, but also the large quantity of data available for analysis made it possible to obtain incidence rates for these reactions in the two sexes separately (MRC Working Party, 1981).

Information concerning adverse reactions was collected in three ways. First, at each follow-up visit, patients were asked if they had been well since the previous appointment, and any symptoms volunteered were noted. No check list of complaints was used. If these complaints were serious enough to justify a change of treatment, whether or not they appeared likely to be drug-related, the co-ordinating centre was notified and, after discussion with the medical staff there, treatment was changed to the alternative active – or placebo – tablets. Second, a self-completed questionnaire listing possible symptoms (modified from Bulpitt & Dollery, 1973) was filled in by each participant. Patients were not withdrawn from randomised treatment on the basis of answers to the questionnaire, though a

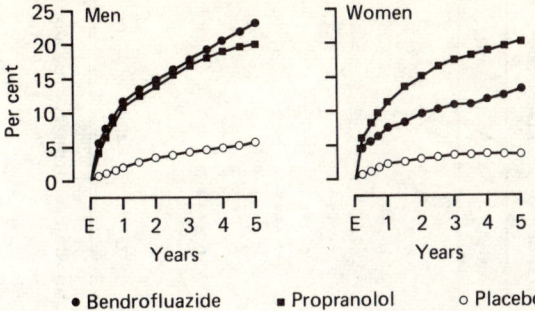

Fig. 6.1. *The proportion of men and women withdrawn from their randomised treatment regime due to adverse drug reactions, according to treatment and time in the trial.*

complaint recorded on a questionnaire might lead to withdrawal if mentioned again at a follow-up visit. Third, routine biochemical investigations sometimes revealed asymptomatic metabolic disturbances, for instance impairment of glucose tolerance, or provided confirmatory evidence of the aetiology of symptoms, for instance showing raised serum uric acid in a patient with joint pains. Biochemical results might thus lead to withdrawal from randomly allocated treatment.

Calculations of the incidence of adverse reactions to the two primary drugs were based on the periods during which these randomly allocated drugs had been used (i.e. either on the total period of observation if a person had remained on his allocated regime, or on the period from starting the drug until its withdrawal, or on the period from starting the drug until the time when supplementary therapy was initiated).

Figure 6.1 shows the proportion of participants withdrawn from randomly allocated treatment due to the development of adverse reactions during their first 5 years in the trial.

The principal clinical reasons for these withdrawals are listed in Table 6.1. The incidence rates of impaired glucose tolerance, lethargy, and constipation, and of nausea, dizziness and headache were significantly increased in both men and women taking bendrofluazide compared with their controls. Men taking bendrofluazide also had a higher incidence of gout (diagnosed on the combination of symptoms and a serum uric acid level exceeding 500 μmol/l) and of impotence, when compared with controls. These two factors largely account for the difference in the rates of withdrawal from bendrofluazide in the two sexes.

Table 6.1. *The principal reasons for withdrawal from randomised treatment in men and women, according to treatment group, numbers of reports and rates/1000 patient-years*[a]

	Men						Women					
	Bendrofluazide		Propranolol		Placebos		Bendrofluazide		Propranolol		Placebos	
	N	rate	N	rate	N	rate	N	rate	N	rate	N	rate
Impaired glucose tolerance	60	7.7***	27	3.4	53	3.3	46	5.9***	16	2.1	31	2.0
Gout[b]	100	12.8***	12	1.5	14	0.9	12	1.5***	—		—	
Impotence	98	12.6***	50	6.3***	20	1.3	—		—		—	
Raynaud's phenomenon	—		41	5.1***	3	0.2	2	0.3	34	4.5***	4	0.3
Skin disorder	6	0.8	12	1.5**	5	0.3	3	0.4	9	1.2**	2	0.1
Dyspnoea	1	0.1	57	7.1***	7	0.4	2	0.3	53	7.1***	3	0.2
Lethargy	28	3.6***	42	5.3***	8	0.5	13	1.7***	62	8.3***	4	0.3
Nausea, dizziness or headache	33	4.2***	33	4.1***	22	1.4	58	7.4***	70	9.4***	27	1.8
Pressure at or above levels requiring change of treatment	8	1.0	33	4.1	611	38.2	11	1.4	24	3.2	400	26.0

[a] Patient-years of observation relates here only to years accrued before withdrawal of randomised treatment and while on primary drug alone.

[b] Defined as symptoms plus serum uric acid in excess of 500 µmol/l in men, 450 µmol/l in women.

** P < 0.01 } Significantly different from rate in controls.
*** P < 0.001

In both sexes propranolol treatment was associated with increased incidence rates of Raynaud's phenomenon, dyspnoea, rashes, lethargy, nausea, dizziness and headache. Some men became impotent while on propranolol.

It is possible that these high rates of adverse reactions would be lower in the context of ordinary practice than in the trial situation where the freedom of choice of drug had been deliberately restricted. Nevertheless the fact that 23% of men on bendrofluazide and 20% of men on propranolol, and 14% of women on bendrofluazide and 21% of women on propranolol, had to be withdrawn from their therapy because one or other of the two most favoured classes of drug for the treatment of mild hypertension caused unacceptable side effects, indicates firstly that prescription needs to be accompanied by careful follow-up, and secondly that the decision to prescribe for any individual with mild hypertension should not be an automatic one.

Unfortunately, the methods of data collection for the course of adverse reactions did not usually allow precise statements to be made of the duration of a reaction after treatment withdrawal. However, it was evident that impotence, developing in association with either active drug, was usually reversible within a few weeks of stopping treatment; about 60% of patients with impaired glucose tolerance while on bendrofluazide had normal glucose tolerance tests within approximately one year of stopping treatment.

Data obtained at interview with the doctor or nurse in a single-blind study may obviously have been selectively reported to the co-ordinating centre; complaints from patients on active drugs were perhaps more likely to be notified than those from people in the placebo group. This problem was discussed extensively at the design stage; the decision to use a single-blind structure was taken because it seemed likely that the general practitioners involved might be unwilling to manage patients in the propranolol group, where individual dosage titration was necessary, without knowing what treatment they were giving. This could have been a serious problem, and concern on this point was strong enough to over-ride worries about the possible bias in reporting. In any case, it seemed unlikely that there would be significant bias affecting the reporting of reactions associated with either drug in comparison with the other, and experience supported this assumption. The association between bendrofluazide and impotence had not previously been established, though that between beta-blocker and impotence was well known. Had reporting been biased, more notifications of the known association than of the unknown one would have been expected, but the reverse was the case: the reported incidence of impotence in men taking bendrofluazide was 3 times greater than that in the propranolol group.

The results obtained from the self-completed questionnaires were of course unaffected by the trial only being single-blind, but the use of the questionnaire was not free of difficulties. It was not clear at first what was the optimum time which should be allowed to elapse between trial entry and filling in the questionnaire which was only done once. Initially this was fixed at 2 years, but because a high proportion of adverse reactions developed after considerably less than this period of exposure the interval was later reduced to 12 weeks. With hindsight, however, it seems that 12 weeks may have been too short an interval: no more than 40% of reports of impotence on bendrofluazide or propranolol, or of Raynaud's phenomenon or dyspnoea on propranolol, were received within the first 3 months of active treatment, though between 70% and 80% occurred within a year of entry, and the questionnaire might have been completed more usefully at the first anniversary of joining the trial. Nonetheless, for easily definable and important reactions such as impotence, dyspnoea, and Raynaud's phenomenon, there was good agreement between the information obtained from questionnaires and at interview, although, possibly because reporting bias was eliminated in the questionnaire data, levels of significance for the comparison between reactions to active and to placebo treatment were lower in this set of results than in those which reached the co-ordinating centre only after assessment by clinic staff. Reporting bias may also have accounted for the difference between interview and questionnaire results for minor complaints, where agreement was less good than for the more major events. Lethargy, for example, was strongly associated, in both men and women, with both active regimes, as judged by the reasons given for withdrawal from randomised treatment; but the results of the questionnaires showed a similar incidence in people taking placebo tablets.

When the trial began, the blood pressure criteria for a change of treatment from placebo tablets to the corresponding active regime were: the development of diastolic pressure (mean of 2 measurements) of 115 mm Hg or more, if confirmed at a further visit 2 weeks later, or the development of systolic pressure of 210 mm Hg or more if similarly confirmed; or the development of pressures of these levels at 3 non-consecutive visits. These criteria were revised (to 110 and 200 mm Hg respectively) in September 1980. It was at about that time that the results of the United States Public Health Service Study (McFate Smith, 1979), the United States Hypertension Detection and Follow-up Program (HDFP) (1979), the Australian National Blood Pressure Study (1980), and the Oslo Study (Helgeland, 1980) were published, and were followed by a number of articles in major medical journals emphasising the benefits due to treatment. An editorial in the New England Journal of Medicine (Relman, 1980) discussing the HDFP results, concluded that 'even patients with diastolic pressures of

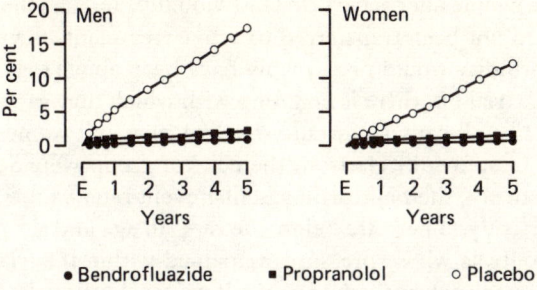

Fig. 6.2. *The proportion of men and women withdrawn from their randomised treatment regime due to blood pressure reaching unacceptable levels, according to treatment and time in the trial.*

90–104 mm Hg will be helped by appropriate drug treatment'. Leading articles in the *British Medical Journal* and the *Lancet* suggested that case detection and treatment of patients with diastolic pressures of 100 mm Hg or more had become mandatory (Anonymous, 1980). The results of the studies and these published recommendations led to a change in the blood pressure criteria which had to be met for a change of trial treatment. Those involved in the scientific and ethical conduct of the trial were not persuaded that the case for active treatment at these lower levels of pressure had been established, but thought that participating doctors, as a result of this increasing external pressure to treat mild hypertensives, might find it difficult to adhere to the original criteria.

Figure 6.2 shows the cumulative proportions of men and women who needed to be withdrawn from randomised treatment because they developed levels of blood pressure above the upper limit for the trial. Of those that completed 5 years in the trial, 18% of men and 13% of women had been transferred from placebo to active drug for this reason. Those overshooting the blood pressure 'ceiling', which defined whether they could remain on their randomised treatment, are shown by sex and treatment regime in Table 6.1. Altogether there were 1011 people (611 men and 400 women) from the untreated control groups who fell into this category. About one-eighth of those entering the control group developed hypertension of a severity which, according to the trial definition, was no longer to be counted as 'mild'. This happened to only 0.4% of those entering the bendrofluazide group and 1.3% of those entering the propranolol group; these people whose pressures were not adequately controlled by the active drugs provided in the trial were withdrawn from their randomly allocated treatment and referred to their own general practitioners for management with other antihypertensive preparations.

Had these people not been treated individually, and had those in the control group not been transferred to active treatment, their cardiovascular morbidity would presumably have been above that of other groups in the trial but there is no group with which they can safely be compared. The all-causes mortality rates of men and women in this category of treated subjects from the control group were 5.7% and 2.9% respectively; their all-cardiovascular event rates were 9.1% and 3.9% respectively. These are below the rates in age and sex matched untreated controls whose pressures remained within the trial range. By continuing to analyse them as controls we are diluting the trial and tending to mask differences between treated and controls. We are thus introducing a bias against a positive result. This is preferable to the omission of such people, as would be the case in 'on treatment' analyses.

Using stepwise multiple logistic regression analyses, the variables which made independent contributions to the probability of exceeding the 'ceiling' limits of pressure were identified in untreated controls. For both sexes, baseline systolic and diastolic pressures made independent positive contributions to the prediction; the independent contribution made by systolic pressure was particularly interesting since in 95% of cases it was the diastolic limit which was exceeded. Age in both men and women made an independent negative contribution, older people being less likely to overshoot the trial blood pressure range.

Table 6.2 shows the rate of overshooting according to various baseline characteristics.

The remaining major reason for withdrawal from randomised treatment was dropping out from follow-up. The overall cumulative loss from the trial, by the end of 5 years, was 19% in both sexes which includes those suffering terminating events and a loss of 3.5% due to participants moving to an area too distant from a trial clinic. The residual 'avoidable' lapse rate, therefore, is 11%. This low figure is a tribute to the good relationships with the patients established by the clinic doctors and nurses. It is also true that the patients valued their participation in the study, feeling that the regular health checks were beneficial.

The total cumulative percentages of men who stopped taking their randomised treatment, including both those withdrawn from their randomly allocated regime but continuing on alternative therapy and routine follow-up and those lapsing from the trial, were 43% of the bendrofluazide group, 42% of the propranolol group, and 47% of the placebo group (Fig. 6.3). Comparable figures for the women were 33%, 40% and 40% respectively. About a third of the men, and almost a third of the women, originally randomised to active treatment, were

Table 6.2. *The characteristics at entry to the trial which made independent contributions to the probability of control subjects exceeding 'ceiling' limits of blood pressure*

	SBP (10 mm Hg increase)	DBP (4 mm Hg increase)	Age (5-year increase)	Female : male	Smokers : non-smokers	Ischaemic ECG : non-ischaemic ECG	Cholesterol (>6.5 : <6.5 mmol/l)	Body mass index (3.0 kg/m² increase)	Tall R waves in left ventr. leads of ECG
P value	<10⁻⁴	<10⁻⁴	<10⁻⁴	<10⁻⁴	0.4	0.4	0.4	1.00	0.006
Relative risk (95% C.I.)	1.25 (1.19–1.32)	1.47 (1.39–1.55)	0.88 (0.83–0.92)	0.59 (0.51–0.68)	1.07 (0.92–1.24)	1.13 (0.86–1.48)	0.94 (0.82–1.08)	1.00 (0.94–1.06)	1.46 (1.13–1.89)

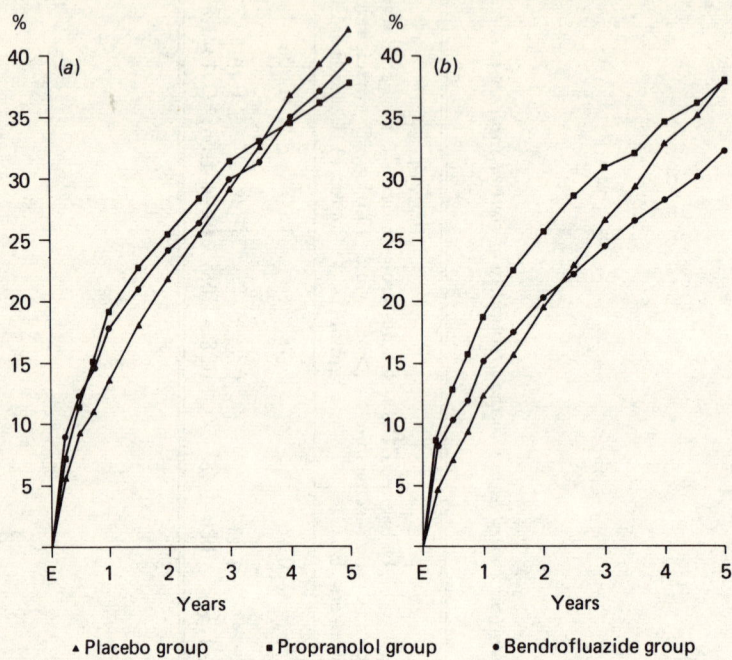

Fig. 6.3a,b. *The proportion of men (a) and women (b) withdrawn from their randomised treatment regime for any reason, according to treatment and time in the trial.*

not being treated with either of the two primary drugs provided by the co-ordinating centre, but many were on other antihypertensive therapy provided by their own doctors. However only about 25% of the person-years of observation of people who should have been on active drugs were lost to the trial and 24% of the person-years of those who should have been on placebo were lost to the trial.

The figures for withdrawals from the trial for the various reasons were high enough to merit examination of their possible effect on the power of the trial and this was carried out some years before the trial ended. The original choice of sample size in the design of the trial had made no specific allowance for the reduction in power due to people withdrawing from their randomised treatment. In the event and after 5 years of follow-up, 15% of those on bendrofluazide and almost 15% of those on propranolol had, at that time, suffered adverse reactions severe enough to require changes of therapy. However, almost all were being managed by interchanging the active regimes; they therefore did not affect the overall comparison of the treated group with the control group. At the time other withdrawals amounted to 4% from terminating events, a 13% drop-out rate from each of the active treatment groups, and a 5% withdrawal from the placebo group due to blood pressures exceeding the ceiling limits. After making various assumptions about the rate at which lapses and terminating events were occurring, for example, and about the rates at which people were developing pressures which exceeded the trial limits, the 'on-treatment' benefit of 40% built into the trial design would be reduced to a benefit of about 37% on an 'as randomised' analysis. The power to detect this as significant at the 1% level overall would decrease from the designed 95% to about 90%.

Such calculations, if they had no other effect, at least reassured the Working Party that they were unlikely to be wasting time and money in pursuing the trial to its planned conclusion.

7 The influences of thiazide and beta-blocker treatment on ECG findings

Electrocardiography was used in the trial as the main objective investigation of the effects of antihypertensive treatment on the heart. Resting ECGs, recorded at entry to the trial and annually thereafter, were read at the co-ordinating centre, without knowledge of the treatment group.

Each ECG was mounted in a re-usable transparent plastic folder. This greatly simplified the handling and reading of ECGs but at its height the trial generated about 17 000 ECGs each year, or about 65 tracings – all to be read twice and some three times – every working day. The task of keeping up to date with ECG reading, and the data processing that went with it, became a chore. Had it been feasible to record electrocardiograms directly on to magnetic tape and have them read by computer, the whole exercise would have been both more efficient and less onerous, but the cost of the recorders for 200 separate clinics would have been prohibitive.

The ECGs were read according to the Minnesota Code which is a coding system used by epidemiologists for recording ECG abnormalities in a standardised way (Rose & Blackburn, 1966). It relies on the accurate observation of heart rates, intervals and amplitudes and the recording of those which satisfy strict criteria for abnormality; the code does not attribute ECG changes to pathological processes.

Each tracing was coded independently by two readers; a third arbitrated when discrepant readings had been recorded. ECG readings in the trial were made without reference to other clinical information, or to previously recorded ECG findings. As the difference between a normal and an abnormal tracing can depend on small differences in amplitudes or intervals, it was not surprising that individuals with ECG characteristics close to the boundaries between normal and abnormal would sometimes be recorded as having a normal and sometimes as having an abnormal reading. In the following analyses we consider only the initial change from 'not having' to 'having' the given abnormality, and ignore any subsequent changes. Only those without the abnormality at entry, and followed up for one or more full years (i.e. with two or more annual ECGs), could be included in analyses of incidence.

The ECG abnormalities were analysed in groups which make clinical sense; for example abnormal Q/QS items, left axis deviation, left ventricular hypertrophy, ST depression with T-wave changes etc. Some people developed more than one of these abnormalities and therefore appear more than once in the tables. This method of dealing with the data seemed better than the alternative of allowing some ECG changes to take precedence over others.

Satisfactory and readable tracings were obtained from almost all participants at entry to the trial; the comparability of the 3 treatment groups at randomisation has already been described. This chapter is concerned with the effects of the thiazide and beta-blocker therapy on the development of ECG abnormalities. The prognostic significance of ECGs in the trial is discussed later.

The significance results quoted below are based on chi-squared tests of the differences between incidence rates at the end of the trial. Probability values are quoted either for all men or all women, or for the two sexes together, and are age-adjusted to correspond with the age structure of the trial population. Nevertheless many comparisons have been made and some 'significant' results are therefore to be expected by chance. The reader should bear this in mind when looking at the values.

Figures 7.1 to 7.3 show the incidence, per 1000 person-years, of certain major groups of abnormalities according to randomised treatment regime and sex. The heights of the columns are proportional to the incidence rates; the numbers on which these figures are based are found in Tables 7.1 to 7.7.

Evidence of transmural infarction

Figure 7.1(a) and Table 7.1 show the incidence of Minnesota Code items 1_1 and 1_2, the more definite manifestations of (or compatible with) transmural myocardial infarction. The overall incidence, for the two sexes together, was reduced in the propranolol group (10.8/ 1000 person-years) compared with controls (12.1/1000 person-years) but the difference was not significant. It was also lower than in the bendrofluazide group (14.2/1000 person-years), and this difference was significant ($P = 0.007$). If the less-definite changes suggesting

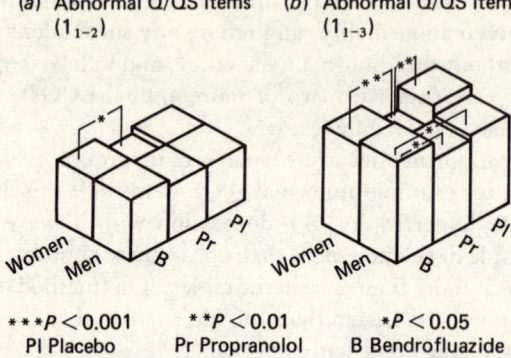

(a) Abnormal Q/QS items (1_{1-2})   (b) Abnormal Q/QS items (1_{1-3})

***$P < 0.001$ **$P < 0.01$ *$P < 0.05$
Pl Placebo   Pr Propranolol   B Bendrofluazide

Fig. 7.1. *The incidence of ECG changes compatible with myocardial infarction, according to randomised treatment regime, in men and women.*

infarction were included (Minnesota Code 1_3) (Fig. 7.1(b)), the reduced overall incidence of abnormal Q/QS complexes of 16.8/1000 person-years in the propranolol group differed significantly from the incidence of 19.8/1000 in the control group ($P = 0.02$); it also differed highly significantly from the rate in the bendrofluazide group of 22.7/1000 person-years ($P = 0.0002$). The overall rate in the thiazide group also differed from the rate in the control group ($P = 0.04$). The data are shown in Table 7.2. An unexplained characteristic of epidemiological studies involving electrocardiog-

Table 7.1. *The incidence of ECG changes compatible with transmural infarction (Minnesota Code 1_{1-2}) according to age, sex and randomised treatment regime. (Rates/1000 person-years of observation)*

Sex	Age	Bendrofluazide		Propranolol		Placebo	
		N	Rate	N	Rate	N	Rate
Men:	35–44	17	9.2	15	7.7	27	7.0
	45–54	48	13.0	50	13.4	92	12.6
	55–64	56	20.0	37	12.5	84	14.5
	Total[a]	121	14.5	102	11.8	203	12.0
Women:	35–44	10	8.4	7	5.7	22	9.6
	45–54	58	18.5	24	7.3	71	11.2
	55–64	40	11.4	47	13.3	101	14.2
	Total[a]	108	13.8+	78	9.7	194	12.3
Both sexes:	Total[a]	229	14.2++	180	10.8	397	12.1

[a] Age-adjusted rates.
Rate differs significantly from propranolol group, ++$P < 0.01$, +$P < 0.05$.

Table 7.2. *The incidence of ECG changes compatible with transmural infarction (Minnesota Code 1$_{1-3}$) according to age, sex and randomised treatment regime. (Rates/1000 person-years of observation)*

Sex	Age	Bendrofluazide		Propranolol		Placebo	
		N	Rate	N	Rate	N	Rate
Men:	35–44	28	15.5	21	11.0	40	10.6
	45–54	83	23.5	67	18.4	139	19.7
	55–64	75	28.0	61	21.6	132	23.8
	Total[a]	186	23.2*[+]	149	17.8	311	19.0
Women:	35–44	22	19.0	8	6.6	35	15.5
	45–54	75	24.7	44	13.9	126	20.6
	55–64	70	21.0	70	20.4	154	22.7
	Total[a]	167	22.2[++]	122	15.7**	315	20.8
Both sexes:	Total[a]	353	22.7*[+++]	271	16.8*	626	19.8

[a] Age-adjusted rates.
Rate differs significantly from control group, **$P < 0.01$, *$P < 0.05$.
Rate differs significantly from propranolol group, [+++]$P < 0.001$, [++]$P < 0.01$, [+]$P < 0.05$.

raphy is the discrepancy between the ECG incidence and the clinical incidence of myocardial infarction in the two sexes (Higgins, Kannel & Dawber, 1965). The similarity in the incidence of ECG evidence of infarction in men and women is well illustrated in these data. The drugs also appear to have a similar influence on these ECG changes in the two sexes.

This overall reduction in the incidence of ECG evidence of infarction in those treated with propranolol, and the marginally increased incidence of such changes in those treated with bendrofluazide, compared with controls, were very interesting findings. So also was the highly significantly greater benefit, in this respect, conferred by propranolol than by bendrofluazide. They are discussed further in Chapter 11, in which the incidence rates of clinical episodes of disease are considered in relation to the type of treatment given.

Left axis deviation

Those treated with propranolol had a reduced incidence of left axis deviation (Minnesota Code 2$_1$) in both sexes. The rate was 27% lower than that in control subjects ($P = 0.005$) and 34% lower than in those on bendrofluazide ($P = 0.0006$). The data are shown in Fig. 7.2(a) and Table 7.3.

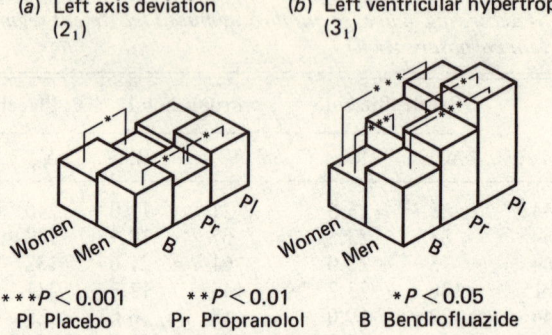

(a) Left axis deviation
    (2_1)

(b) Left ventricular hypertrophy
    (3_1)

*** $P < 0.001$ ** $P < 0.01$ * $P < 0.05$
Pl Placebo   Pr Propranolol   B Bendrofluazide

Fig. 7.2. *The incidence of left axis deviation, and of left ventricular hypertrophy, according to randomised treatment regime, in men and women.*

Table 7.3. *The incidence of left axis deviation (Minnesota Code 2_1) according to age, sex and randomised treatment regime. (Rates/1000 person-years of observation)*

Sex	Age	Bendrofluazide		Propranolol		Placebo	
		N	Rate	N	Rate	N	Rate
Men:	35–44	16	8.8	9	4.7	21	5.5
	45–54	37	10.4	28	7.7	91	13.1
	55–64	44	16.5	34	12.5	80	14.9
	Total[a]	97	12.1[+]	71	8.7*	192	12.0
Women:	35–44	9	7.7	6	4.9	7	3.0
	45–54	29	9.3	17	5.2	35	5.6
	55–64	41	12.4	28	8.3	87	12.8
	Total[a]	79	10.4[+]	51	6.5	129	8.4
Both sexes:	Total[a]	176	11.3[+++]	122	7.6**	321	10.2

[a] Age-adjusted rates.
Rate differs significantly from control group, ** $P < 0.01$, * $P < 0.05$.
Rate differs significantly from propranolol group, [+++] $P < 0.001$, [+] $P < 0.05$.

Left ventricular hypertrophy

As would be expected the development of the amplitude criteria for LVH (Minnesota Code 3_1), in those who entered the trial without this abnormality, was reduced in people randomised to receive active drugs compared with placebo ($P < 0.0001$). Both bendrofluazide and propranolol conferred benefit in this respect, but in every age group of both sexes (Table 7.4) the incidence of LVH, as defined, was reduced in the bendrofluazide group to a greater extent than in the

Table 7.4. *The incidence of left ventricular hypertrophy (Minnesota Code 3.1)*
according to age, sex and randomised treatment regime. (Rates/1000 person-years
of observation)

Sex	Age	Bendrofluazide		Propranolol		Placebo	
		N	Rate	N	Rate	N	Rate
Men:	35–44	26	14.6	36	19.9	63	17.3
	45–54	43	12.3	58	16.3	171	25.3
	55–64	44	16.5	52	19.5	133	24.8
	Total[a]	113	14.2***	146	18.2*	367	23.3
Women:	35–44	9	7.7	13	10.7	23	10.3
	45–54	28	9.0	51	16.2	87	14.1
	55–64	34	10.0	57	16.8	173	26.1
	Total[a]	71	9.3***+++	121	15.6	283	18.9
Both sexes:	Total[a]	184	11.8***+++	267	16.9**	650	21.1

[a] Age-adjusted rates.
Rate differs significantly from control group, ***$P < 0.001$, **$P < 0.01$, *$P < 0.05$.
Rate differs significantly from propranolol group, +++$P < 0.001$.

propranolol group (Fig. 7.2(b)). The overall reduction in incidence
was 44% for the thiazide group and 20% for the beta-blocker group;
this difference between the two active drug groups was also significant
($P = 0.0002$).

Multiple regression analysis was carried out to determine whether
the reduced incidence of LVH in the treated subjects, and the greater
reduction in those on the thiazide than in those on the beta-blocker,
were explained by the differences between the groups in the levels of
their treated blood pressures. Correcting for the differences between
groups in their blood pressures as recorded at the 6-month follow-up
visit reduced the significance of the difference in the incidence of
amplitudes suggesting LVH between treated and control subjects,
and also that between those on bendrofluazide and propranolol, but in
neither case did it abolish it; both these differences remained significant ($P < 0.001$). This suggests perhaps, that there may be a
metabolic effect of the thiazide added to its hypotensive effect in
reducing the incidence of LVH.

ECG changes of LVH and strain were relatively infrequent in the
mild hypertensives in the MRC trial (Table 7.5). The incidence of
such changes (defined in Minnesota Code terms as 3_1 with 4_{1-3} and
5_{1-2}) was also reduced in those on active drugs compared with placebo
and the 47% reduction in those randomised to bendrofluazide was
again significantly different from the 30% reduction in the propranolol
group.

Table 7.5. *The incidence of left ventricular hypertrophy and strain (Minnesota Code 3_1 with 4_{1-3}, 5_{1-2}) according to age, sex and randomised treatment regime. (Rates/1000 person-years of observation)*

Sex	Age	Bendrofluazide		Propranolol		Placebo	
		N	Rate	*N*	Rate	*N*	Rate
Men:	35–44	1	0.5	1	0.5	5	1.3
	45–54	7	1.8	5	1.3	16	2.1
	55–64	8	2.7	10	3.3	25	4.2
	Total[a]	16	1.9	16	1.8	46	2.6
Women:	35–44	1	0.8	1	0.8	3	1.3
	45–54	3	0.9	3	0.9	6	0.9
	55–64	4	1.1	11	3.0	32	4.4
	Total[a]	8	1.0*	15	1.8	41	2.5
Both sexes:	Total[a]	24	1.4*	31	1.8	87	2.6

[a] Age-adjusted rates.
Rate differs significantly from control group, *$P < 0.05$.

Abnormalities of repolarisation

The effects of the two primary regimes on the repolarisation of the myocardium were different in the two sexes (Table 7.6). In women the incidence of ST depression with T-wave changes (4_{1-3} with 5_{1-3}) was increased (by 45%) in those on bendrofluazide compared with controls ($P < 0.0001$) and by 58% compared with those on propranolol ($P < 0.0001$). The relative increase was greatest in younger women. Propranolol had little effect on ST/T wave changes in women (Fig. 7.3(a)). Among men the thiazide was not associated with a high incidence of ST/T wave changes, but propranolol reduced the rate compared with controls ($P = 0.0001$) and with men on bendrofluazide ($P = 0.002$). The sexes also responded differently to the two primary drug regimes in terms of T-wave changes which were not accompanied by ST changes (5_{1-3}) (Table 7.7 and Fig. 7.3(b)). In women but not in men the incidence of T-wave abnormalities was increased in those on both the thiazide and the β-blocker ($P = 0.004$ and 0.01 respectively) whereas in men the thiazide was associated with a significant reduction in such abnormalities, compared with control subjects ($P = 0.001$).

A multiple regression analysis was carried out to determine whether the increased incidence of repolarisation abnormalities in women in the thiazide group was explained by hypokalaemia. A significant

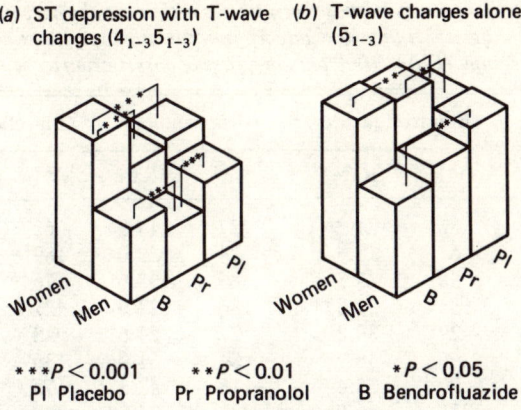

(a) ST depression with T-wave changes ($4_{1-3}5_{1-3}$)

(b) T-wave changes alone (5_{1-3})

***$P < 0.001$ **$P < 0.01$ *$P < 0.05$
Pl Placebo   Pr Propranolol   B Bendrofluazide

Fig. 7.3. *The incidence of abnormalities of repolarisation of the myocardium, according to randomised treatment regime, in men and women.*

Table 7.6. *The incidence of repolarisation abnormalities – ST depression accompanied by T-wave inversion (Minnesota Code 4_{1-3}, 5_{1-3}) according to age, sex and randomised treatment regime. (Rates/1000 person-years of observation)*

Sex	Age	Bendrofluazide		Propranolol		Placebo	
		N	Rate	N	Rate	N	Rate
Men:	35–44	10	5.5	10	5.1	29	7.5
	45–54	50	13.6	30	8.1	107	14.8
	55–64	79	29.5	54	19.2	156	28.5
	Total[a]	139	17.1[++]	94	11.1***	292	17.7
Women:	35–44	31	27.8	6	4.9	24	10.7
	45–54	89	30.8	59	18.9	125	20.7
	55–64	109	35.4	90	27.3	185	27.8
	Total[a]	229	32.4***[+++]	155	20.5	334	22.4
Both sexes:	Total[a]	368	24.2**[+++]	249	15.6**	626	19.9

[a] Age-adjusted rates.
Rate differs significantly from control group, ***$P < 0.001$, **$P < 0.01$.
Rate differs significantly from propranolol group, [+++]$P < 0.001$, [++]$P < 0.01$.
Trends differ in the two sexes.

Table 7.7. *The incidence of repolarisation abnormalities – T-wave changes in the absence of ST segment changes (Minnesota Code 5_{1-3}) according to age, sex and randomised treatment regime. (Rates/1000 person-years of observation)*

Sex	Age	Bendrofluazide		Propranolol		Placebo	
		N	Rate	N	Rate	N	Rate
Men:	35–44	36	21.2	27	14.9	62	17.2
	45–54	61	18.5	74	22.0	189	29.1
	55–64	58	25.5	85	35.6	176	37.8
	Total[a]	155	21.3**	186	24.6	427	29.0
Women:	35–44	29	30.2	27	24.6	38	18.6
	45–54	96	38.9	84	31.0	136	25.2
	55–64	90	35.4	116	42.3	196	34.4
	Total[a]	215	36.0**	227	34.8*	370	28.1
Both sexes:	Total[a]	370	27.9	413	29.4	797	28.6

[a] Age-adjusted rates.
Rate differs significantly from control group, ** $P < 0.01$, * $P < 0.05$.
Trends differ in the two sexes.

relationship was found between serum potassium level and repolarisation abnormalities in the thiazide-treated women and correcting for the minimum potassium value recorded during the follow-up removed the highly significant difference in such abnormalities between women in the bendrofluazide and control groups. It also reduced the significance of the difference between the incidence of 5_{1-3} codes in women on bendrofluazide and in controls from $P < 0.01$ to $P < 0.05$.

Abnormalities of rhythm

Abnormalities of rhythm were infrequent with the exceptions of sinus bradycardia and sinus tachycardia which were both common. Sinus bradycardia, which was induced by propranolol, and sinus tachycardia which was inhibited by propranolol, showed very different rates in the treatment groups. Atrial fibrillation and flutter, A–V nodal rhythm, ventricular tachycardia and supraventricular tachycardia were all too infrequent to allow analysis of any influence of the trial drugs on their incidence.

Ventricular and supraventricular extrasystoles, however, were sufficiently common to merit analysis. The incidence of ventricular ectopic arrhythmias had, in fact, been monitored from an early stage of the follow-up. Ventricular and supraventricular extrasystoles are codable under the Minnesota Code if they occur at a frequency of 10%

Table 7.8. *The incidence of ECG supraventricular ectopic arrhythmias (Minnesota Code $8_{1(S)}$) according to age, sex and randomised treatment regime. (Rates/1000 person-years of observation)*

Sex	Age	Bendrofluazide		Propranolol		Placebo	
		N	Rate	N	Rate	N	Rate
Men:	35–44	2	1.1	4	2.0	2	0.5
	45–54	7	1.8	7	1.8	15	2.0
	55–64	23	7.9	15	4.9	30	5.0
	Total[a]	32	3.7	26	2.9	47	2.7
Women:	35–44	1	0.8	1	0.8	2	0.9
	45–54	5	1.5	3	0.9	10	1.5
	55–64	14	3.9	5	1.4	34	4.6
	Total[a]	20	2.5	9	1.1**	46	2.8
Both sexes:	Total[a]	52	3.1	35	2.0	93	2.8

[a] Age-adjusted rates.
Rate differs significantly from control group, **$P < 0.01$.

or more of all beats. Table 7.8 shows the incidence of supraventricular ectopic arrhythmias to be significantly reduced in women on propranolol compared with female controls ($P < 0.01$); there is no similar trend among men. Table 7.9 shows the incidence of ventricular ectopic arrhythmias, as so defined. Overall, the reduced rate for those on propranolol differed from that of those on bendrofluazide

Table 7.9. *The incidence of ventricular ectopic arrhythmias (Minnesota Code $8_{1(V)}$) according to age, sex and randomised treatment regime. (Rates/1000 person-years of observation)*

Sex	Age	Bendrofluazide		Propranolol		Placebo	
		N	Rate	N	Rate	N	Rate
Men:	35–44	7	3.7	8	4.1	13	3.3
	45–54	17	4.5	13	3.4	42	5.6
	55–64	33	11.5	19	6.3	55	9.3
	Total[a]	57	6.7	40	4.5	110	6.4
Women:	35–44	8	6.7	4	3.2	10	4.3
	45–54	11	3.4	21	6.3	25	3.9
	55–64	30	8.4	14	3.8	45	6.1
	Total[a]	49	6.1	39	4.7	80	4.9
Both sexes:	Total[a]	106	6.4+	79	4.6	190	5.7

[a] Age-adjusted rates.
Rate differs significantly from propranolol group, +$P < 0.05$.

($P = 0.04$). Neither rate differed significantly from that in controls but at an earlier stage in the trial's follow-up the incidence of ventricular ectopic arrhythmias in men treated with bendrofluazide had been found to be significantly ($P < 0.01$) higher than in control men. This earlier observation had been made at a time when the incidence of trial terminating events for coronary heart disease was running at a higher rate in the bendrofluazide group of men than in controls.

These two observations tended to confirm reports linking thiazide treatment with cardiac arrhythmias (Holland, Nixon & Kuthnert, 1981; Hollifield & Slaton, 1980) and led to a sub-study within the MRC trial in which 24-h ambulatory cardiography was carried out in trial participants receiving either bendrofluazide or placebo therapy. This sub-study was undertaken by Dr Paul Whelton, a visiting American research fellow. It was a good example of the value of the general practice research framework in providing an opportunity to investigate, on a large scale, a problem which was not common, and to compare findings with those in matched controls drawn from the same populations. Its detailed results have been published (MRC Working Party, 1983).

The study had two parts. One involved 110 new trial entrants who were randomly assigned one of three treatments: bendrofluazide with potassium supplements, bendrofluazide without potassium supplements, or placebo. They were studied by 24-h ambulatory ECG monitoring, routine resting ECGs and serum biochemistry before starting treatment and 9–10 weeks later while still taking their assigned drugs. No significant increase in the number of ventricular extrasystoles resulted from this short-term thiazide treatment although the serum potassium concentrations became higher with the potassium supplements and lower in those on bendrofluazide alone.

In the other part of the study, 214 people who had completed an average of two years's treatment with randomly assigned bendrofluazide (95 subjects) or placebo (99 subjects) had 24-h ECG monitoring, a routine ECG and serum biochemical tests while continuing to take their trial tablets. The 214 also included 20 people who had been specially selected because at some stage they had developed hypokalaemia. These 20 patients were studied before and 5 weeks after being further randomised to either a continuation of bendrofluazide unchanged or to a continuation of bendrofluazide but with potassium supplementation.

In this part of the study ventricular ectopic beat counts were found to be significantly higher ($P < 0.025$) in those receiving long-term thiazide treatment than in their age- and sex-matched controls (Fig. 7.4). This finding in a group whose mean serum potassium level was

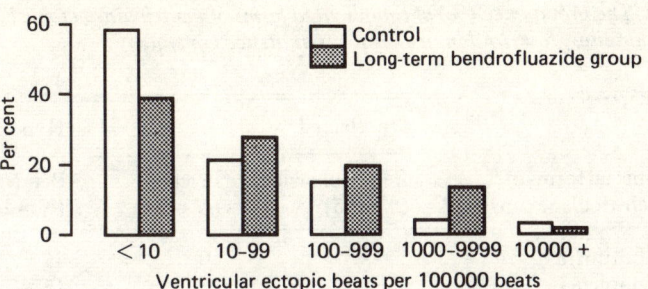

Fig. 7.4. *The distribution of ventricular ectopic beat counts in 24-h ECGs in a long-term thiazide group, and in age- and sex-matched controls.*

3.6 mmol/l, in comparison with that of 4.1 mmol/l in controls, was therefore consistent with the published work. But no convincing evidence could be found of a simple causative relationship between low concentrations of serum potassium and high ventricular ectopic beat counts. The short-term study of new entrants taking unsupplemented thiazide showed that they experienced the expected fall in serum potassium levels but no increase in ventricular extrasystoles; those taking potassium-supplemented thiazide, despite a small drop in serum potassium levels, showed significantly lower ectopic beat counts. No relationship between changes in serum potassium level and changes in ectopic beat count could be demonstrated in any part of the study, and although giving supplementary potassium to the hypokalaemic group increased their serum potassium levels it had no effect on their 24-h ectopic beat counts.

Only by pooling data from the various groups in the sub-study was it possible to show a significant relationship between ectopic beat counts and serum potassium levels. In fact they were significantly ($P = 0.003$) but weakly, correlated ($r = -0.185$). The degree of correlation between serum potassium levels and ectopic beats was matched, almost exactly, by a significant ($P = 0.004$) positive correlation ($r = 0.178$) between serum urate levels and ectopic beats. There was no clinical reason for suspecting that serum urate levels influenced ectopic activity (though it is a risk factor for coronary heart disease) and serum urate levels were chosen for analysis only to demonstrate that the relationship between ventricular ectopic arrhythmias and thiazide use could be due to any of the biochemical changes which occur with thiazides; both serum potassium levels and serum urate could have been acting merely as markers of thiazide intake. The causative factor could be the serum potassium level; it could equally be some other change resulting from thiazide ingestion, such as magnesium depletion.

Table 7.10. *The prevalence (%) of complicated forms of ventricular ectopic beats in long-term thiazide group and in age- and sex-matched controls*

Special forms of ventricular extrasystoles	Unselected		Hypokalaemic
	Bendrofluazide (N = 95)	Placebo (N = 99)	Bendrofluazide (N = 20)
Multiform	17	10	35
Couplets	5	2	15
R on T beats	9	1	10
Bigeminy	7	1	5

The clinical significance of modest differences in ventricular ectopic beat counts remains unclear. But one aspect of this study caused some concern. The prevalence of complicated forms of ectopic beat – multifocal extrasystoles, couplets, R on T forms and bigeminy – was higher in long-term thiazide takers than in their placebo controls, and higher still among those selected as having been hypokalaemic (Table 7.10). Nevertheless the MRC Working Party believed that unless the postulated relationship between thiazide intake and ventricular ectopic arrhythmias was manifest in terms of mortality or morbidity, the trial should proceed unchanged, and the protocol was not changed in this respect.

The relationship between cigarette smoking, thiazide and beta-blocker treatment, and ECG changes

Figures 7.5(a) and 7.5(b) show, for both sexes together, the incidence of the groups of Q/QS abnormalities shown in Fig. 7.1; the incidences of LAD and LVH are shown for smokers and non-smokers in Fig. 7.6(a) and 7.6(b); the relation between smoking and repolarisation abnormalities, which showed a marked sex difference in incidence, is shown for the two sexes separately in Figs. 7.7 and 7.8.

Within treatment groups, cigarette smoking seemed to bear little overall relationship to the incidence of ECG changes of possible myocardial infarction (Figs. 7.5(a) and 7.5(b)). This was surprising in view of the very clear-cut relationships in both sexes between smoking and the incidence of cardiovascular, especially coronary, complications.

Between treatment groups there was no overall difference in the incidence of abnormal Q/QS items among smokers; the difference in

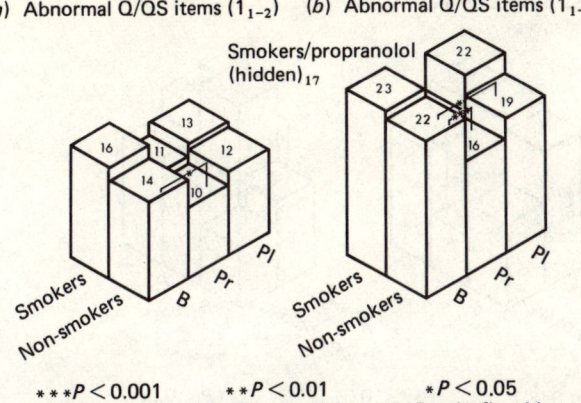

(a) Abnormal Q/QS items (1_{1-2})   (b) Abnormal Q/QS items (1_{1-3})

Smokers/propranolol (hidden)$_{17}$

Smokers

Non-smokers

B   Pr   Pl

$***P < 0.001$ $**P < 0.01$ $*P < 0.05$
Pl Placebo   Pr Propranolol   B Bendrofluazide

Fig. 7.5. *The incidence of ECG changes compatible with myocardial infarction in smokers and non-smokers according to randomised treatment regime; both sexes together.*

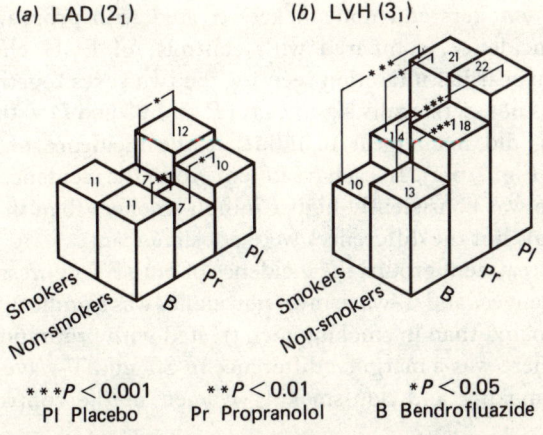

(a) LAD (2_1)   (b) LVH (3_1)

Smokers

Non-smokers

B   Pr   Pl

$***P < 0.001$ $**P < 0.01$ $*P < 0.05$
Pl Placebo   Pr Propranolol   B Bendrofluazide

Fig. 7.6. *The incidence of left axis deviation and of left ventricular hypertrophy in smokers and non-smokers according to randomised treatment regime; both sexes together.*

(a) ST depression and T-wave   (b) T-wave inversion
changes

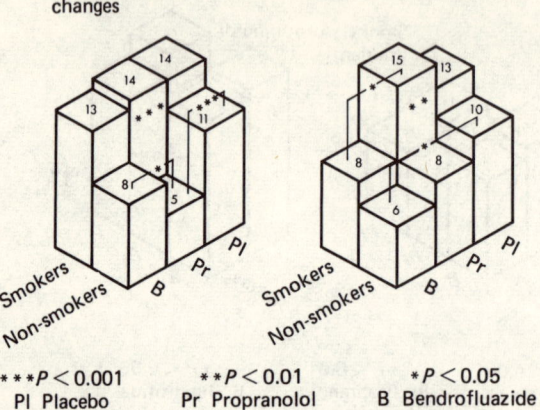

***P < 0.001   **P < 0.01   *P < 0.05
Pl Placebo   Pr Propranolol   B Bendrofluazide

Fig. 7.7. *The incidence of abnormalities and repolarisation in smoking and non-smoking men according to randomised treatment regime.*

incidence of both the more definite abnormalities (1.1 and 1.2 codes) and the total Q/QS items (1.1–3 codes) between the two active treatment groups did not quite achieve statistical significance, $P = 0.06$ in each case. In non-smokers the total incidence of such changes (Fig. 7.5(b)) was reduced in the propranolol group and the difference from the rate in non-smokers on bendrofluazide was highly significant ($P = 0.0005$). However, the rate in the non-smokers was higher in those on bendrofluazide than in controls ($P = 0.03$).

In both smokers and non-smokers treated with propranolol the reduced incidence, compared with controls, of ECG changes of possible myocardial infarction seen for the two sexes together (Fig. 7.4(b)) was not statistically significant ($P = 0.08$ and $P = 0.07$).

Smoking did not appear to influence the incidence of left axis deviation (Fig. 7.6(a). In each treatment group the incidence of LVH amplitudes was consistently higher in non-smokers than in smokers (Fig. 7.6(b)) but the differences were not significant.

Within treatment groups the incidence of both ST depression with T-wave changes, and T-wave inversion alone, was significantly lower in non-smoking than in smoking men treated with propranolol (Fig. 7.7) and there was a marginal difference in ST and T-wave changes between smoking and non-smoking women in the control group (Fig. 7.8).

Between treatment groups the differences were found largely in non-smokers in both sexes and they again differed between the two sexes. The incidence of ST and T-wave changes was reduced in men on propranolol, compared with both the thiazide ($P < 0.05$) and the

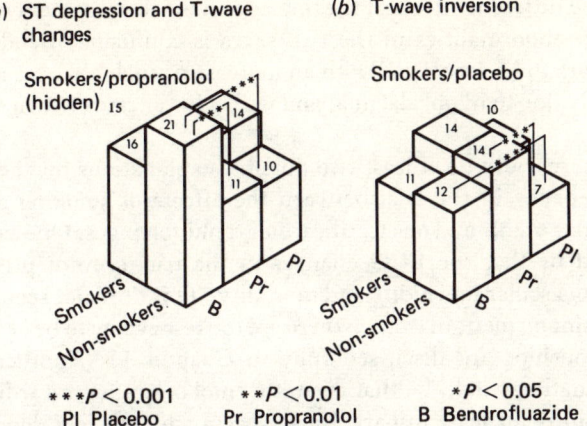

(a) ST depression and T-wave changes

(b) T-wave inversion

*** P < 0.001   Pl Placebo   ** P < 0.01   Pr Propranolol   * P < 0.05   B Bendrofluazide

Fig. 7.8. *As for Fig. 7.7, but for women.*

control group ($P = 0.0001$) (Fig. 7.7(a)), and was increased in women on bendrofluazide compared with controls ($P < 0.0001$) or compared with those on propranolol ($P < 0.0001$) (Fig. 7.8(a)). These sex differences, previously mentioned above, seem to be present only in non-smokers.

The incidence of T-wave inversion was higher in smoking than non-smoking men treated with propranolol, but otherwise apparently not influenced by smoking habit in either sex.

Summary of ECG incidence results

Perhaps the most important finding in this analysis of electro-cardiographic changes resulting from treatment with thiazide and β-blockers is the significantly reduced incidence of ECG evidence of myocardial infarction in those treated with propranolol, compared with untreated controls (Table 7.2). Also of interest was the apparently increased rate of abnormal Q/QS items in those on the thiazide compared with controls.

As a consequence of these two trends (each of which was statistically significant but not highly so) propranolol treatment produced an incidence rate of Q/QS items (1_{1-3}) which was highly significantly reduced compared with the rate in the thiazide group. The analysis also showed propranolol to be more effective than bendrofluazide in preventing left axis deviation, and markedly less effective in preventing the development of LVH.

The different effects of the thiazide on the development of repolarisation abnormalities in the two sexes is confusing. Bendrofluazide appears to be associated with an increase of such changes in women, largely due to hypokalaemia, and with a lower rate of such changes in men.

There could be at least two possible explanations for the apparent discrepancy in the trial between the effects of smoking on cardiovascular events and on electrocardiographic changes. One explanation would be that the ECG changes in the trial are not predictive of cardiovascular morbidity and mortality. This does not seem to be the case among men; in women there are too few events to be certain. The relationships are discussed fully in Chapter 11. Another possible explanation would be that cigarette smoking induces cardiovascular morbidity, at least in part, by a process which is less dependent on coronary atheroma and ECG changes. Epidemiological studies on coagulation factors have shown that smoking is associated with raised plasma fibrinogen levels ($P < 0.001$) (Meade, 1984) and raised plasma fibrinogen levels significantly predict increased coronary mortality (Meade *et al.*, 1986).

Between-drug differences in the incidence of Q/QS items and repolarisation abnormalities were found to be greater in non-smokers than smokers. Several of these features are supported by similar relationships between drug treatment and CHD events, discussed in Chapter 11.

8 The monitoring of trial-terminating events

The trial's end-points were deaths from any cause, non-fatal myocardial infarctions and non-fatal strokes. When news of a possible terminating event reached the practice, the trial nurse notified the co-ordinating centre using the form illustrated in Fig. 8.1.

Letters were sent where appropriate to hospital records departments, to consultants, to coroners and to general practitioners asking for detailed histories of each episode and a résumé of the clinical findings, including pathology reports, electrocardiograms, the results of enzyme tests etc. The evidence concerning each episode was willingly provided and usually wholly adequate. It was assessed by a single observer (Professor Hugh Tunstall Pedoe) who was kept unaware of the treatment the individual had been receiving.

Once terminating events had begun to build up in number, assessments were carried out every 3 months, and the results were plotted on a series of sequential analysis charts. Three sets of primary analyses were carried out:

(1) All-causes mortality
(2) Fatal and non-fatal stroke, combined
(3) All cardiovascular-renal deaths and events.

For each of these primary analyses, charts were kept comparing all treated with all control subjects for the two sexes together and for each sex separately. Similar sets of charts compared events in the two active treatment groups, as randomised, and each separate treatment group with controls. Because uncertainty also existed about the benefits from treatment for other groups of events, the monitoring of myocardial infarction deaths, and of all coronary deaths and events (including sudden deaths) was also undertaken. The Monitoring Committee recognised that the interpretation of conventional levels of statistical significance would be influenced by the multiplicity of combinations of end-points which were under observation, but believed it essential that the co-ordinating centre should monitor for effects which could be important even though they were not anticipated in the original design of the trial.

NO CARBON
REQUIRED

MRC TREATMENT TRIAL FOR MILD HYPERTENSION

NOTIFICATION OF TERMINATING EVENT

NAME .... NUMBER [ ][ ][ ][ ][ ][ ][ ]   1- 8

CARD No.   [6][0]   9-10

DATE OF NOTIFICATION OF TERMINATING EVENT   [ ][ ][ ]   11-16
                                          Day Month Year

This patient has been withdrawn from the trial due to:-

NON-FATAL MYOCARDIAL INFARCTION   Y or N [ ]   17

   If 'Yes', date of infarction   [ ][ ][ ]   18-23
                                          Day Month Year

   Was patient admitted to hospital?   Y or N [ ]   24

     If 'Yes', which hospital? ....

     Under which consultant? ....

     If 'No', please give name and address of practitioner from whom
       further details could be obtained

        ....

        ....

NON-FATAL CEREBROVASCULAR ACCIDENT   Y or N [ ]   37

   If 'Yes', date of CVA   [ ][ ][ ]   38-43
                                          Day Month Year

   Was patient admitted to hospital?   Y or N [ ]   44

     If 'Yes', which hospital? ....

     Under which consultant? ....

     If 'No', please give name and address of practitioner from whom
       further details could be obtained

        ....

        ....

DEATH   Y or N [ ]   57

   If 'Yes', date of death   [ ][ ][ ]   58-63
                                          Day Month Year

Place of death ....

Was death sudden (i.e. within 24 hrs of onset of symptoms)?   Y or N [ ]   64

Please give certified cause of death

    Ia ....

     b ....

     c ....

    II ....

Was an autopsy performed?   Y or N [ ]   65

Signed ....

PLEASE DETACH TOP COPY AND POST TO MRC/DHSS EPIDEMIOLOGY AND MEDICAL CARE UNIT, NORTHWICK PARK HOSPITAL, WATFORD ROAD, HARROW, MIDDLESEX HA1 3UJ

Fig. 8.1. *The form used for the notification of terminating events.*

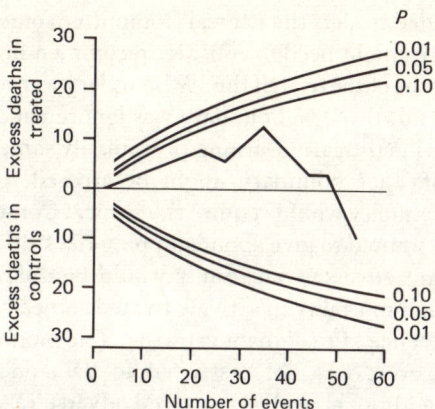

Fig. 8.2. *The type of chart used for sequential analyses (hypothetical data).*

Sequential charts, of the type illustrated with hypothetical data in Fig. 8.2, were examined by members of the Monitoring Committee and by the chairman of its Ethical Committee every 3 months. Although the charts were updated quarterly, significance testing was carried out less often. The position of the boundaries corresponding with 10%, 5% and 1% statistical significance had been calculated on the basis of a total of 15 statistical tests spread over the duration of the trial; significance testing was carried out annually in December 1975, December 1976 and December 1977 and thereafter every 6 months for a further 6 years. Thus although the charts were scrutinised every 3 months no notice was taken of a boundary being crossed if this occurred at a time when statistical testing was not due. On the occasions when the charts were subject to statistical testing, copies were also sent to all members of the Ethical Committee.

The adoption of an early warning system

The monitoring of beneficial and of adverse effects of the trial was carried out separately and for each an early warning system was devised. This alerted the ethical committee of a trend at a stage which would allow time for full consideration, and if necessary further analyses, before any recommendation to discontinue the study might need to be made. For an adverse effect of the trial, where one or both treatment groups were faring less well than control subjects, or one active treatment group was faring less well than the other, the crossing of the 10% significance boundary was taken as the early warning signal; this was intended to alert the Ethical Committee some months before the event that it might need to consider recommending termination of the trial, or part of the trial, if the 5% boundary were crossed.

For a beneficial trend, the 10% boundary was ignored and the 5% boundary would provide the early warning presumably some months before the 1% significance boundary might be crossed. Only the crossing of the 1% boundary would require the Ethical Committee to decide what advice it wanted to give about stopping the study.

The most important adverse trial results would be unfavourable trends in morbidity and mortality in actively treated subjects, including an increased incidence of malignant growths. The monitoring of adverse effects, however, was not restricted to data on primary terminating events; additional analyses covered adverse reactions to trial drugs (see Chapter 6) and the incidence of such secondary trial end-points as congestive cardiac failure, angina pectoris, or the development of ECG evidence of myocardial infarction. Such events could lead to the withdrawal of a subject from his or her randomised treatment, but were not counted as terminating events.

The definition of trial-terminating events

(1) All-causes mortality

The death of a person attending regularly for trial follow-up was usually known by the clinic and transmitted to the co-ordinating centre. The name, address and NHS number of anyone whose continued follow-up at a trial clinic had stopped, for whatever reason, were notified to those keeping the central register of the National Health Service at Southport. The co-ordinating centre would then be informed if such a subject died or emigrated.

The certified cause of death was reviewed by the trial's independent arbiter in the light of all available clinical and autopsy information. Occasionally, but rarely, the cause of death as certified was judged to be incorrect and reclassified; it must be stressed that the arbiter did not know the treatment or placebo status of the individual.

(2) All cardiovascular–renal deaths and events

This classification of terminating events included deaths from hypertensive heart and renal disease (ICD 400–404), deaths from cerebrovascular disease (ICD 430–438), deaths from ischaemic heart disease (ICD 410–414), sudden death of unknown cause occurring within one hour of the onset of symptoms and a group of other relevant deaths including dissecting aneurysm, congestive cardiac failure, left ventricular failure, peripheral vascular disease, arterial embolism and cardiomyopathy. The classification also included non-fatal cerebrovascular accidents, excluding transient ischaemic attacks; and nonfatal episodes of myocardial infarction.

(3) Stroke

Stroke was defined as a rapidly developing episode with clinical signs of focal or global disturbance of cerebral function lasting for more than 24 h, with no apparent cause other than a vascular one. This is the definition adopted by the World Health Organisation (Aho, Harmsen, Hatano *et al.*, 1980).

(4) Myocardial infarction

This was also defined according to WHO criteria (World Health Organisation, 1976). Definite myocardial infarction was diagnosed when there were unequivocal serial ECG changes, a typical or atypical history with definitely raised enzyme levels and equivocal ECG changes, a typical history with raised enzymes alone, or post mortem appearances of fresh myocardial infarction and/or coronary occlusion at autopsy. Possible myocardial infarction was diagnosed in living patients on the basis of a typical history (provided there was no good evidence of another diagnostic cause) without definite ECG or enzyme confirmation, and in fatal cases with a past history of ischaemic heart disease or autopsy evidence of chronic occlusion or stenosis or old myocardial scarring (provided, again, that there was no good evidence of another cause of death). The analyses of coronary events described later include definite and possible MI categories combined.

The effects of prolonged recruitment on trial monitoring

Recruitment of the first patient to enter the pilot trial took place in March 1973 but for reasons already given the last did not join the study until February 1982. Thus there were many participants who had completed their $5\frac{1}{2}$ years before others had entered the trial. From the start the system of monitoring terminating events had been to record them on the sequential analysis charts as they were assessed. This meant that events were recorded without regard to the duration of the person's participation in the trial. This system would be satisfactory if there were no relationship between the time since entry to the trial and the occurrence of the event, but if there were such a relationship this could be concealed by the way the data were handled. For the reasons described in Chapter 9, from December 1980 a set of sequential charts showing events plotted according to the time interval since entry to the trial was computed after each assessment session.

9 The effects of treatment on trial morbidity and mortality

On 9 June, 1983, the routine assessment of trial-terminating events met one of the primary criteria on which the Ethical Committee would be asked to advise on the trial's future. Sequential analysis showed an overall reduction in strokes, significant at the 1% level, in men and women randomised to active treatment compared with controls.

As is happened the 'early warning system' – which had been devised to allow time and opportunity for the Ethical Committee to obtain further analyses, if necessary, before having to advise on the continuation of the trial – was short-circuited by a run of 12 strokes (one in a treated person and 11 in control subjects). This had taken the sequential plot in one step from a point between the 10% and 5% significance boundaries across the 1% significance line (Fig. 9.1).

Under its terms of reference the Ethical Committee was required to alert the Secretary of the Council (Sir James Gowans) and the Chairman of the Working Party (Professor W. S. Peart) if the Committee were satisfied that (in either both sexes combined or in one sex) a difference between treated and control subjects was significant at the 1% level in one of the following: (a) total mortality; (b) stroke mortality and stroke morbidity; or (c) cardiovascular mortality and morbidity. The Ethical Committee was also asked to advise on whether the trial, having reached such a result, should be terminated and if so, whether the termination should affect selected age groups or the whole trial.

On 7 July the Chairman of the Ethical Committee (Sir Richard Doll) duly alerted those concerned that the 1% boundary had been crossed for stroke, but nevertheless recommended that the trial should be continued. The trial had reached a position where, in terms of its overall results, it had demonstrated benefit in one class of cardiovascular complications, at a time when the effect on total mortality was slightly but not significantly, adverse. The reduction in stroke rate, therefore, had to be balanced against possible adverse effects on other event rates. As the results at that stage provided no clear guidance on the overall value of treating people with mild

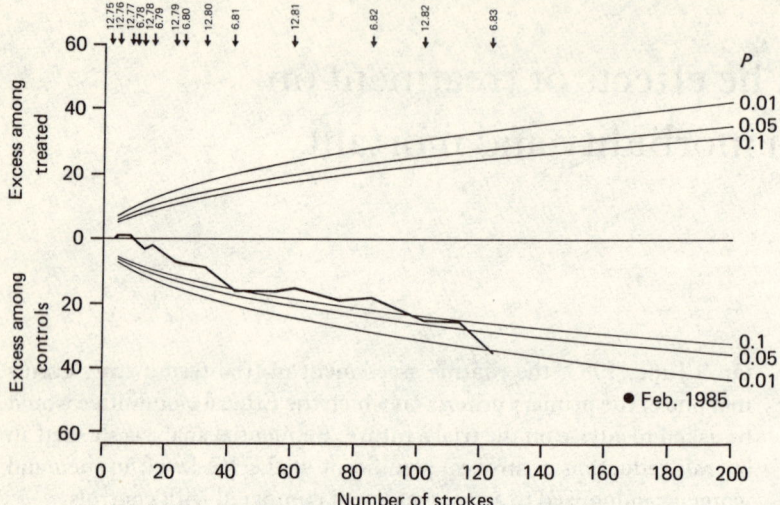

Fig. 9.1. *Sequential analysis chart for stroke comparing treated with controls; both sexes together. (The use of such charts was discontinued from June 1983: the positions of the plots by February 1985 are shown for interest only.)*

hypertension, and as there were already grounds for believing that its further prolongation might provide useful information on sub-groups, the trial was continued. The only major sub-group analysis that had been considered at that time was that of cigarette smokers and non-smokers. It is discussed in Chapter 10.

In recommending the continuation of the trial the Ethical Committee had asked the Monitoring Committee to report on analyses (which were already in progress) of the interaction between smoking and the type of antihypertensive drug administered in determining cardiovascular event rates, and to continue to report on the overall results at 6-monthly intervals. This was done and the trial continued until the end of February, 1985 by which time the main results were as described below.

Stroke

During the course of the trial to February, 1985, 169 strokes had occurred, 102 in men and 67 in women. Sixty were in people to whom active drugs had been allocated and 109 were in control subjects (Table 9.1). This 45% reduction in the overall stroke incidence rate

Table 9.1. Strokes and stroke rates/1000 person-years of observation according to age, sex and randomised treatment regime

Sex	Age	Treated						Controls	
		Bendrofluazide		Propranolol		Active drugs[b]		Placebo	
		N	Rate	N	Rate	N	Rate	N	Rate
Men:	35–44	—	0.0	3	1.2	3	0.6	2	0.4
	45–54	2	0.4	9	1.9	11	1.1	23	2.4
	55–64	9	2.4	14	3.7	23	3.1	40	5.3
	Total[a]	11	1.0***+	26	2.3	37	1.7**	65	2.9
Women:	35–44	1	0.6	2	1.2	3	0.9	5	1.6
	45–54	2	0.5	4	0.9	6	0.7	11	1.3
	55–64	4	0.9	10	2.2	14	1.5	28	3.1
	Total[a]	7	0.7**	16	1.5	23	1.1*	44	2.1
Both sexes:	Total[a]	18	0.8***+++	42	1.9	60	1.4***	109	2.6

[a] Age-adjusted rates.
[b] Those randomised to either bendrofluazide or propranolol.
Rate differs significantly from control group ***$P < 0.001$, **$P < 0.01$, *$P < 0.05$.
Rate differs significantly from propranolol group ++$P < 0.01$, +$P < 0.05$.

from 2.6 to 1.4 per thousand person-years of observation (which had been significant at the 1% level on sequential analysis 20 months previously) was now very highly significant on one-off testing ($P = 0.0006$). The benefit was shared between the sexes – 43% in men, 48% in women – and was present in all 3 decades of age at entry to the trial. In the 35–44, 45–54 and 55–64 age groups reductions in stroke rates were from 0.9 to 0.7/1000 person-years (15%), from 1.9 to 0.9/1000 person-years (51%), and from 4.1 to 2.2/1000 person-years (46%) respectively.

When analysed according to entry diastolic pressure expressed in intervals of 5 mm Hg – below 95, 95–99, 100–104, and 105 mm Hg and over – the stroke incidence in untreated controls increased from one group to the next – 1.4, 2.3, 3.1 and 4.4/1000 person-years, respectively (Table 9.2). But the percentage benefits of treatment were irregular; reductions in stroke rates in those on active treatment were 40%, 18%, 50% and 69% respectively. However, absolute benefits (differences between control and treated rates) tended to increase progressively (0.6, 0.5, 1.5 and 3.0 strokes per 1000 person-years, respectively). Table 9.3 shows strokes and stroke rates in those with entry pressures above and below 100 mm Hg. For those with diastolic pressures of 100–109 mm Hg, the reduction in stroke rate from 3.6 to 1.5/1000 person-years was 59%, and was recorded in both active drug groups (bendrofluazide – 72%, propranolol – 48%) and in both sexes (men – 50%, women – 72%) (Tables 9.4 and 9.5). Among those on active treatment with diastolic pressures at entry of 90–99 mm Hg, the overall reduction in stroke rate was from 1.8 to 1.4/1000 person-years. The benefit conferred by bendrofluazide was present in both groups; that associated with propranolol seemed only to exist in those with entry pressures above 100 mm Hg (Table 9.3).

Forty-five strokes were fatal, 124 non-fatal. Bendrofluazide was associated with a 70% reduction in fatal strokes and a 65% reduction in non-fatal strokes; propranolol with a 2% increase in fatal and a 32% reduction in non-fatal strokes. Unfortunately and due to a mistake in the design of the record booklet, information on transient ischaemic attacks (which were defined as episodes in which a focal neurological deficit of less than 24-h duration occurred) was recorded in the same 'box' as that used for vaso-vagal attacks. It was impossible to differentiate between responses to questions concerning these two conditions.

The overall benefit conferred by treatment with bendrofluazide appeared to differ from that due to propranolol. Of the 60 strokes which occurred among those who had been randomised to active drugs, 18 were in the thiazide group and 42 in the beta-blocker group. The difference in stroke rates between the two groups had not been

Table 9.2. *Strokes and stroke rates/1000 person-years of observation according to age, entry diastolic pressure and randomised treatment regime. Both sexes together*

| | Treated | | | | | | Controls | |
| | Bendrofluazide | | Propranolol | | Active drugs[a] | | Placebo | |
DBP (V) (mm Hg)	N	Rate	N	Rate	N	Rate	N	Rate
<95	1	0.2	9	1.5	10	0.8	17	1.4
95–99	8	1.3	16	2.4	24	1.8	29	2.3
100–104	5	1.0	11	2.2	16	1.6	32	3.1
105+	4	1.1	6	1.6	10	1.4	31	4.4

[a] Those randomised to either bendrofluazide or propranolol.

Table 9.3. *Strokes and stroke rates/1000 person-years of observation, in those with entry diastolic pressures above or below 100 m Hg, according to age and randomised treatment regime. Both sexes together.*

Entry pressure DBP (V) (mm Hg)	Age	Treated						Controls	
		Bendrofluazide		Propranolol		Active drugs[b]		Placebo	
		N	Rate	N	Rate	N	Rate	N	Rate
<100	35–44	1	0.4	1	0.4	2	0.4	2	0.4
	45–54	1	0.2	9	1.7	10	0.9	15	1.4
	55–64	7	1.5	15	3.1	22	2.3	29	3.0
	Total[a]	9	0.7*+	25	2.0	34	1.4	46	1.8
100+	35–44	–	0.0	4	2.3	4	1.2	5	1.6
	45–54	3	0.9	4	1.1	7	1.0	19	2.7
	55–64	6	1.7	9	2.6	15	2.1	39	5.6
	Total[a]	9	1.0***	17	1.9*	26	1.5****	63	3.6
90–109	Total[a]	18	0.8****++	42	1.9	60	1.4****	109	2.6

[a] Age-adjusted rates.
[b] Those randomised to either bendrofluazide or propranolol.
Rate differs significantly from control group rate ***$P < 0.001$, **$P < 0.01$, *$P < 0.05$.
Rate differs significantly from propranolol group rate ++$P < 0.01$, +$P < 0.05$.

Table 9.4. *Strokes and stroke rates/1000 person-years of observation, in those with entry diastolic pressures above or below 100 m Hg, according to age and randomised treatment regime. Men.*

Entry pressure DBP (V) (mm Hg)	Age	Treated						Controls	
		Bendrofluazide		Propranolol		Active drugs[b]		Placebo	
		N	Rate	N	Rate	N	Rate	N	Rate
<100	35–44	—	0.0	1	0.7	1	0.3	—	0.0
	45–54	—	0.0	7	2.4	7	1.2	10	1.6
	55–64	4	1.9	7	3.1	11	2.5	20	4.6
	Total[a]	4	0.6*+	15	2.2	19	1.4	30	2.2
100+	35–44	—	0.0	2	1.9	2	1.0	2	1.0
	45–54	2	1.1	2	1.0	4	1.0	13	3.8
	55–64	5	3.2	7	4.7	12	3.9	20	6.4
	Total[a]	7	1.5*	11	2.5	18	2.0*	35	4.0
90–109	Total[a]	11	1.0***+	26	2.3	37	1.7**	65	2.9

[a] Age-adjusted rates.
[b] Those randomised to either bendrofluazide or propranolol.
Rate differs significantly from control group rate *** P < 0.001, ** P < 0.01, * P < 0.05.
Rate differs significantly from propranolol group rate + P < 0.05.

Table 9.5. *Strokes and stroke rates/1000 person-years of observation, in those with entry diastolic pressures above or below 100 m Hg, according to age and randomised treatment regime. Women.*

Entry pressure DBP (V) (mm Hg)	Age	Treated						Controls	
		Bendrofluazide		Propranolol		Active drugs[b]		Placebo	
		N	Rate	N	Rate	N	Rate	N	Rate
<100	35–44	1	1.1	—	0.0	1	0.5	2	1.1
	45–54	1	0.4	2	0.8	3	0.6	5	1.0
	55–64	3	1.2	8	3.0	11	2.1	9	1.7
	Total[a]	5	0.8	10	1.7	15	1.3	16	1.3
100+	35–44	—	0.0	2	2.9	2	1.5	3	2.4
	45–54	1	0.6	2	1.1	3	0.9	6	1.7
	55–64	1	0.5	2	1.0	3	0.8	19	4.9
	Total[a]	2	0.5**	6	1.3	8	0.9**	28	3.3
90–109	Total[a]	7	0.7***	16	1.5	23	1.1*	44	2.1

[a] Age-adjusted rates.
[b] Those randomised to either bendrofluazide or propranolol.
Rate differs significantly from control group rate **$P < 0.01$, *$P < 0.05$.

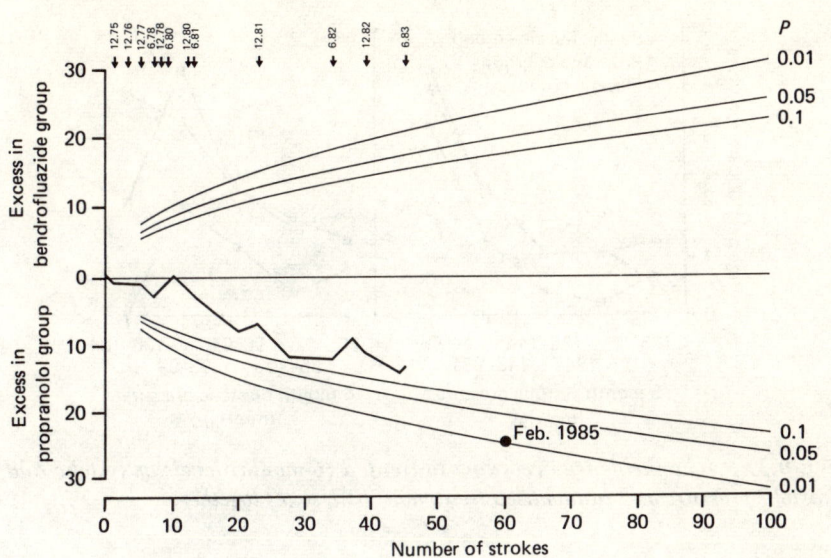

Fig. 9.2. *Sequential analysis chart for stroke comparing bendrofluazide with propranolol groups; both sexes together.*

significant on sequential testing by June, 1983 (Fig. 9.2) but became significant ($P = 0.002$) on the basis of a one-off look at the time the trial was stopped in February, 1985.

It is possible that the better blood pressure control achieved by treatment with bendrofluazide compared with propranolol (described in Chapter 5) may have contributed to the lower stroke incidence in the thiazide group especially as the difference in blood pressure control was greatest in the older subjects. Of the strokes, 156 (92%) occurred in people over the age of 45 at entry to the trial. Figure 9.3 shows stroke incidence according to levels of systolic and diastolic pressure while under treatment. At each level of both systolic and diastolic pressure as recorded at the examination undertaken 6 months after entry, the stroke incidence was lower in the bendrofluazide group than in the propranolol group. This suggests that the thiazide confers some benefit, in terms of stroke, over and above that attributable to its effect in lowering blood pressure. The size of the benefit also suggests that bendrofluazide may have prevented cerebral infarction as well as cerebral haemorrhage. It would seem important to confirm this in other studies and to attempt to explain it. One possibility, quite speculative, would be that seemingly equivalent levels of pressure resulting from the action of a beta-blocker with its reduction of catecholamine activity, and from a thiazide diuretic are not physiologically comparable. The near superimposition of the curves relating

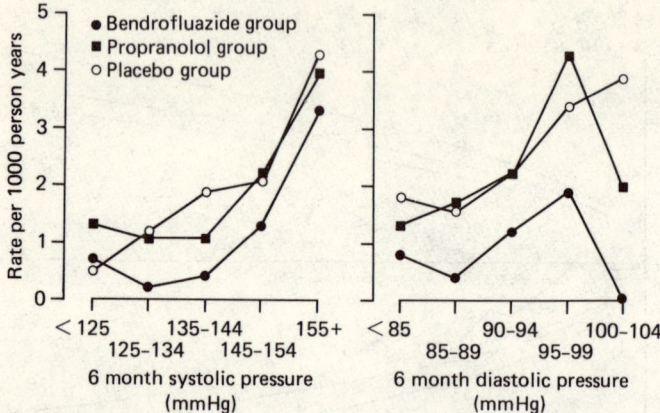

Fig. 9.3. *Stroke incidence according to treated (6-month) levels of systolic and diastolic pressure and randomised treatment; both sexes together.*

stroke incidence with 6-month systolic and diastolic pressures in the propranolol and control groups suggests that the stroke benefit associated with propranolol is explained entirely by its effects on blood pressure levels.

Myocardial infarction, including sudden death

At the time of the assessment of trial events in February 1985, 456 MIs or sudden cardiac deaths had occurred. Of these, 384 were in men and 72 in women; 222 were in people randomised to active treatment and 234 in controls (Table 9.6). These figures, and the sequential plot showing the occurrence of events up to June 1983 (Fig. 9.4), indicate that the trial regimes had no *overall* effect on the incidence of myocardial infarction.

Of the 456 terminating coronary events, 203 (45%) were fatal. In the bendrofluazide group there were 59 fatal MIs, a 22% increase compared with controls, whereas in the propranolol group there were 47 fatal MIs, a 5% reduction. For all MIs, fatal and non-fatal, the thiazide group showed a 2% increase, the propranolol group a 13% reduction. None of these differences was significant but the situation by the time the trial ended masked trends which at an earlier phase had caused anxiety to those monitoring the trial.

Sequential analysis charts comparing MI incidence in those on bendrofluazide with those on propranolol are shown for men and

Table 9.6. *All coronary events and rates/1000 person-years of observation, according to age, sex and randomised treatment regime*

Sex	Age	Treated				Active drugs[b]		Controls	
		Bendrofluazide		Propranolol				Placebo	
		N	Rate	N	Rate	N	Rate	N	Rate
Men:	35–44	11	4.4	10	3.9	21	4.2	17	3.3
	45–54	33	6.9	39	8.0	72	7.5	83	8.7
	55–64	55	14.9	36	9.6	91	12.2	100	13.4
	Total[a]	99	9.0	85	7.6	184	8.3	200	9.0
Women:	35–44	1	0.6	1	0.6	2	0.6	1	0.3
	45–54	7	1.7	5	1.2	12	1.4	9	1.1
	55–64	12	2.6	12	2.6	24	2.6	24	2.6
	Total[a]	20	1.9	18	1.7	38	1.8	34	1.7
Both sexes:	Total[a]	119	5.6	103	4.8	222	5.2	234	5.4

[a] Age-adjusted rates.
[b] Those randomised to either bendrofluazide or propranolol.

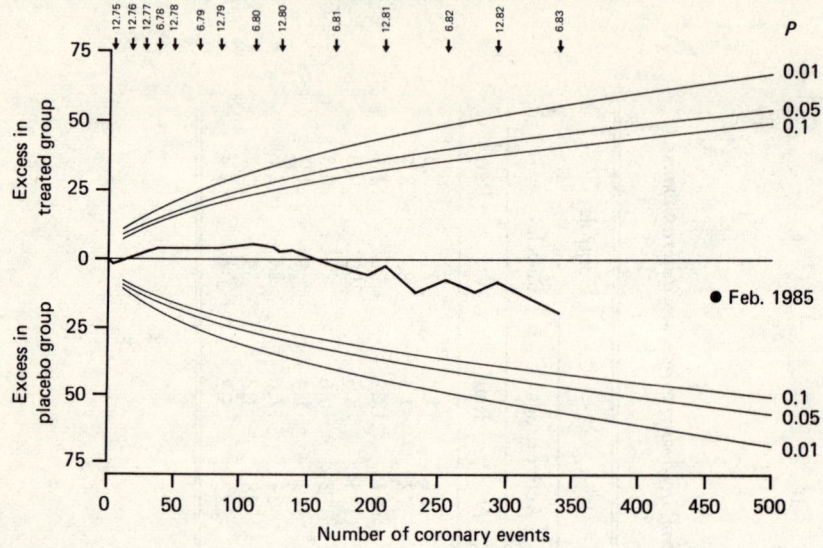

Fig. 9.4. *Sequential analysis chart for coronary events comparing treated with controls; both sexes together.*

women for the period to June 1983 in Figs. 9.5 and 9.6. In men the excess of events in the thiazide group had twice crossed the 10% significance boundary and once reached the 5% line; subsequent results changed the course of the plot and the final was well within the 10% boundary. In women the excess of MI events occurred in those randomised to propranolol; the sequential plot had also crossed the 10% boundary and closely approached the 5% significance line before later events changed its course and the final point was far from either 10% boundary line.

These trends, occurring in a classification of terminating events (fatal and non-fatal MI plus sudden deaths) which had not been designated initially as a separate group for sequential analysis, led to a series of unsuccessful attempts to explain them. The apparent excess of MIs in men on thiazide seemed unrelated to any of the biochemical changes being monitored. In particular low serum potassium levels were not encountered any more frequently in those suffering MIs than in a comparison group.

But the trial was not well designed for this kind of investigation because biochemical measurements were carried out only at annual medical examinations and for an individual the time interval between the event and the most recent biochemical profile could be up to one year. Likewise the apparent excess of MIs did not appear to be due to

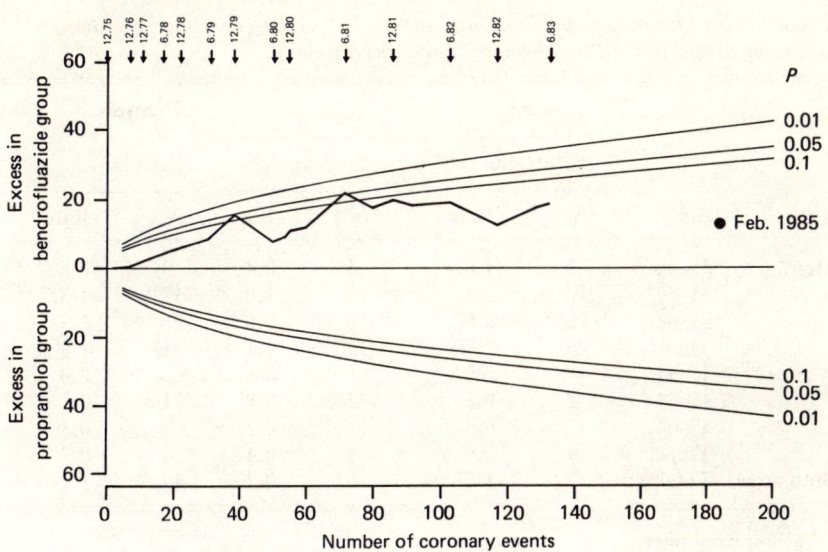

Fig. 9.5. *As for Fig. 9.4, but comparing bendrofluazide with propranolol groups; men.*

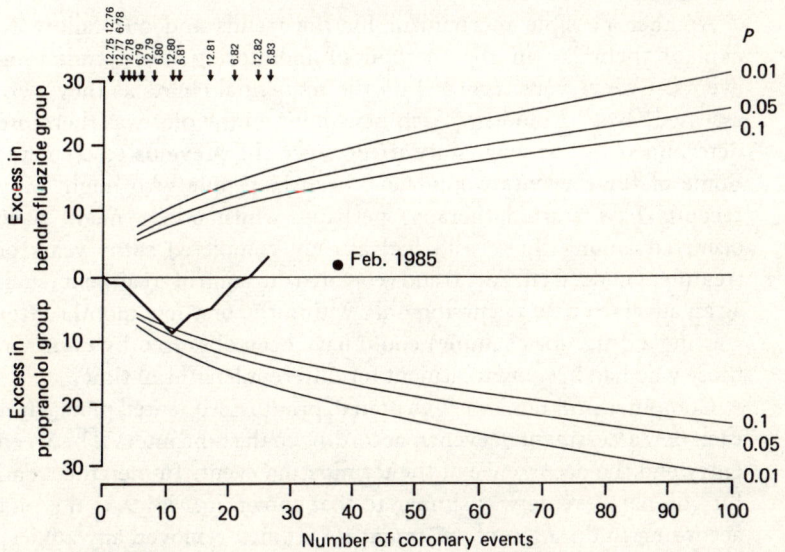

Fig. 9.6. *As for Fig. 9.5, but for women.*

Table 9.7. *Sudden coronary deaths, and rates/1000 person-years of observation, according to age, sex and randomised treatment regime*

| | | Treated | | | | Controls | |
| | | Bendrofluazide | | Propranolol | | Placebo | |
Sex	Age	N	Rate	N	Rate	N	Rate
Men:	35–44	4	1.6	1	0.4	3	0.6
	45–54	12	2.5	5	1.0	12	1.3
	55–64	13	3.6	6	1.6	26	3.5
	Total[a]	29	2.7[++]	12	1.1	41	1.9
Women:	35–44	–	0.0	1	0.6	–	0.0
	45–54	2	0.5	2	0.5	1	0.1
	55–64	2	0.4	1	0.2	3	0.3
	Total[a]	4	0.4	4	0.4	4	0.2
Both sexes:	Total[a]	33	1.6[+]	16	0.7	45	1.1

[a] Age-adjusted rates.
Rate differs significantly from propranolol group rate [++]$P = 0.01$, [+]$P < 0.05$.

less-adequate blood pressure control, or to drug-induced hypotension, nor was it associated either with ECG abnormalities present at entry to the trial or with ECG abnormalities developing subsequently. The reason for the early excess of coronary events in women on propranolol also remained obscure. The trends in both sexes may have been due to chance.

Another possible mechanism for the trends and our failure to explain them lay in the method of monitoring trial-terminating events. Events were recorded on the sequential charts as they were assessed, every 3 months. Each new point on the plot was therefore determined by the events occurring since the previous assessment. Some of these events would have been in people who might only recently have started therapy, perhaps, whilst others might have occurred among those who had already completed some years of treatment in the trial. Any trend related to duration of treatment (such as an adverse effect occurring only within the first few months after starting a drug, for example) could have been obscured by events in those who had been on treatment for different lengths of time.

Computer programs were written to produce sequential plots, after each new assessment of events, according to the time interval between entry and the occurrence of the terminating event. In men the trend for coronary events was similar to that shown in Fig. 9.5; the plot according to duration of treatment for women removed any anxiety about a possible adverse effect of propranolol.

Sudden death was defined as death occurring within one hour of the onset of symptoms, and was assumed to be due to coronary heart

Table 9.8. *Fatal coronary events, and sudden deaths, occurring in men within their first year in the trial, according to randomised treatment regime. N and rate/1000 person-years*

	Bendrofluazide		Propranolol		Placebo	
	N	Rate	N	Rate	N	Rate
Fatal CHD events	9	4.0	3	1.3	11	2.4
Sudden deaths	6	2.7	–	0.0	3	0.7

disease unless an autopsy showed some other cause. Ninety-four (46%) of the 203 fatal coronary events were judged to be sudden deaths. The data are shown in Table 9.7. There were 29 sudden deaths in men in the thiazide group (2.7 per 1000 person-years), 12 in men in the propranolol group (1.1 per 1000 person-years) and 41 in male controls (1.9 per 1000 person-years); the difference between the two active drug groups is significant for men alone ($P = 0.01$) and for the two sexes together ($P = 0.02$); the differences between those on active treatment and untreated controls were not significant.

The incidence of fatal coronary events and sudden deaths in men according to their year in the Trial (Table 9.8) shows suggestive evidence that the coronary benefit from propranolol, and the possible coronary hazard from the thiazide, are concentrated in the first year of treatment. The differences however were not statistically significant.

The recognition of a possibly adverse effect of thiazide on coronary events, especially on fatal coronary events, though not statistically significant, was nevertheless sufficiently worrying for the Chairman of the trial's Ethical Committee to advise the Working Party to consider halving the dose of the thiazide used. A special meeting of the Working Party was convened but it was decided not to alter the treatment of those already in the trial. To act in a way which might condemn a class of drugs which were so valuable and in such world-wide use could only be justified on the strongest of evidence, and the trial results were not conclusive. To change the regime in mid-trial would have removed the chance to answer this important question.

Although it was decided not to change the dose for those already on the thiazide – which would have caused widespread repercussions – it was agreed to try to get better evidence about the value of different doses of the drug, with and without potassium supplements, in those still to be recruited into the trial. The results of this factorially designed sub-study are discussed in Chapter 12.

The relationships found in the trial between coronary events, antihypertensive treatment and cigarette smoking are discussed in Chapter 10.

Table 9.9. All cardiovascular events and rates/1000 person-years of observation, according to age, sex and randomised treatment regime

Sex	Age	Treated						Controls	
		Bendrofluazide		Propranolol		Active drugs[b]		Placebo	
		N	Rate	N	Rate	N	Rate	N	Rate
Men:	35–44	11	4.4	13	5.1	24	4.8	19	3.7
	45–54	37	7.8	48	9.9	85	8.8	108	11.3
	55–64	65	17.6	51	13.6	116	15.6	145	19.4
	Total[a]	113	10.3	112	10.0	225	10.2*	272	12.3
Women:	35–44	2	1.3	3	1.9	5	1.6	6	2.0
	45–54	9	2.2	9	2.1	18	2.2	20	2.4
	55–64	16	3.5	22	4.7	38	4.1	54	5.9
	Total[a]	27	2.6	34	3.2	61	2.9	80	3.9
Both sexes:	Total[a]	140	6.6*	146	6.7*	286	6.7**	352	8.2

[a] Age-adjusted rates.
[b] Those randomised to either bendrofluazide or propranolol.
Rate differs significantly from control group **$P < 0.01$, *$P < 0.05$.

Table 9.10. *All deaths and all-causes mortality/1000 person-years of observation, according to age, sex and randomised treatment regime*

| | | Treated | | | | Controls | | | |
| | | Bendrofluazide | | Propranolol | | Active drugs[b] | | Placebo | |
Sex	Age	N	Rate	N	Rate	N	Rate	N	Rate
Men:	35–44	8	3.2	7	2.7	15	3.0	11	2.1
	45–54	29	6.1	27	5.5	56	5.8	64	6.7
	55–64	45	12.2	41	10.9	86	11.6	106	14.2
	Total[a]	82	7.5	75	6.7	157	7.1	181	8.2
Women:	35–44	2	1.3	3	1.9	5	1.6	5	1.6
	45–54	16	3.9	17	4.0	33	3.9	24	2.9
	55–64	28	6.1	25	5.4	53	5.7	43	4.7
	Total[a]	46	4.5	45	4.3	91	4.4	72	3.5
Both sexes:	Total[a]	128	6.0	120	5.5	248	5.8	253	5.9

[a] Age-adjusted rates.
[b] Those randomised to either bendrofluazide or propranolol.

All cardiovascular terminating events

The great majority of cardiovascular terminating events resulted from either myocardial infarction or stroke; partly due to the definition of a terminating event, and partly due to the age range observed in the study, less than 2% of all cardiovascular events were attributed to other causes.

By the end of the trial, 638 cardiovascular events had occurred – 497 in men and 141 in women. Among the actively treated 286 occurred, and in controls, 352 (Table 9.9). This represented an overall reduction of 19% which on 'one off' testing at the end of the trial was significant ($P = 0.01$). This overall benefit was shared between the sexes – 17% in men, 25% in women. For the two sexes together the overall benefit was very similar for each primary drug – a 20% reduction on bendrofluazide and an 18% reduction on propranolol.

Total mortality

During the course of the trial 501 deaths occurred, 338 in men, 163 in women (Table 9.10). All-cause mortalities were almost identical in the treated and control groups – 248 and 253 deaths respectively giving rates of 5.8 and 5.9 per 1000 person-years. The 248 deaths in those on active treatment were shared almost equally between the thiazide (128) and the propranolol groups (120).

The all-cause mortality rates were apparently affected differently by active treatment in the two sexes. In men there were 157 deaths on active treatment and 181 on placebo – a 13% reduction; among women there were 91 deaths in the actively treated and 72 in those on placebo – a 25% increase. The difference between the sexes in this respect was marginally significant ($P = 0.05$).

10 The influence of cigarette smoking on trial morbidity and mortality

Trial participants were questioned about their smoking habits when they entered the trial and at each of the annual medical examinations thereafter. Had the crucial importance of the information about smoking been appreciated from the outset, different questions would have been asked, but for simplicity they had been restricted to 'Do you smoke cigarettes now?' and if so 'How many a day?' Thus no information was obtained about pipe or cigar smokers and it was impossible to distinguish them from non-smokers; likewise it was impossible to distinguish ex-smokers from those who had never smoked.

About 30% of men, and 25% of women, were smokers of cigarettes at entry to the trial. These were low proportions compared with the national figures at that time, and accord with the concept that the trial participants were rather more 'health conscious' than average men and women. Tables 10.1 and 10.2 show comparisons of the characteristics of smokers and non-smokers in the two sexes at entry, according to their randomised treatment regime. No important differences were apparent between treatment groups in either sex, but within each group there were significant differences between smokers and non-smokers, some of which were expected, others not.

Among men the cigarette-smokers were somewhat younger, had faster pulse rates, were lighter in weight and had lower values of serum urea and serum uric acid levels (possibly due to dietary differences) than the non-smokers. There were no significant differences in serum cholesterol levels between smokers and non-smokers and – probably due to the constraints on the range of blood pressures of those admitted to the study – no significant differences in their mean systolic or diastolic pressures. Among women the cigarette smokers weighed less and had lower serum urea levels than the non-smokers but did not differ significantly in blood pressures, pulse rates, serum uric acid or cholesterol values.

Table 10.1. *The comparability of smokers and non-smokers at entry to the trial. Men*

Entry characteristics	Smokers			Non-smokers		
	Bendrofluazide group (N = 706)	Propranolol group (N = 691)	Placebo group (N = 1423)	Bendrofluazide group (N = 1517)	Propranolol group (N = 1579)	Placebo group (N = 3091)
Mean age (y)	50.2	50.0*	49.8***	50.7	50.7	51.0
Mean systolic pressure (mm Hg)	158.2	158.9	158.7	157.4	157.9	157.9
Mean diastolic pressure (mm Hg)	98.0	98.1	97.9	98.3	98.5	98.1
Mean pulse rate/min	82.0***	81.7***	81.7***	79.2	79.4	79.2
Mean weight (kg)	79.5***	80.2**	79.4***	82.4	82.0	82.0
Mean serum cholesterol (mmol/l)	6.3	6.2	6.2	6.3	6.3	6.2
Mean serum urea (mmol/l)	5.1***	5.1***	5.1***	5.5	5.5	5.5
Mean serum uric acid (μmol/l)	374.6***	367.6***	365.6***	385.3	376.6	377.1
% abnormal Q-wave items	3.1	1.3	1.4	0.9	1.1	1.6
% ST-T wave abnormalities	0.6*	0.7	1.3	1.7	1.1	1.0
% Past history of treatment for hypertension	4.7	3.5	4.1	5.1	4.2	4.0
% Past history of stroke	1.1	0.9	0.8	0.7	0.6	0.6
% Past history of myocardial infarction	0.8	0.9	0.6	1.0	0.8	0.9

Value in smokers significantly different from that in non-smokers ***$P < 0.001$, **$P < 0.01$, *$P < 0.05$.

Table 10.2. *The comparability of smokers and non-smokers at entry to the trial. Women*

Entry characteristics	Smokers			Non-smokers		
	Bendrofluazide group (N = 555)	Propranolol group (N = 537)	Placebo group (N = 1108)	Bendrofluazide group (N = 1499)	Propranolol group (N = 1570)	Placebo group (N = 3002)
Mean age (y)	52.3	52.7	52.3*	52.8	52.7	52.8
Mean systolic pressure (mm Hg)	164.7	165.5	165.3	165.4	165.5	165.1
Mean diastolic pressure (mm Hg)	98.2	98.7	98.7	98.6	98.6	98.3
Mean pulse rate/min	82.9	83.1	83.4	83.4	83.3	83.3
Mean weight (kg)	68.8**	67.7***	68.1***	70.7	70.5	70.4
Mean serum cholesterol (mmol/l)	6.6	6.7	6.7	6.7	6.6	6.7
Mean serum urea (mmol/l)	5.0****	4.9****	5.0****	5.2	5.2	5.2
Mean serum uric acid (μmol/l)	293.5	291.8	292.6	298.0	294.0	293.4
% abnormal Q-wave items	2.2	1.1	1.4	1.6	1.7	1.4
% ST-T wave abnormalities	2.3	1.3	1.5	2.0	1.3	1.8
% Past history of treatment for hypertension	11.0	11.0	10.4	10.4	12.0	11.0
% Past history of stroke	0.4	6.9	0.5	0.9	0.7	0.8
% Past history of myocardial infarction	0.2	0.4	0.3	0.0	0.2	0.1

Value in smokers significantly different from that in non-smokers *** $P < 0.001$, ** $P < 0.01$, * $P < 0.05$.

122

Table 10.3. *All deaths and all-causes mortality/1000 person-years of observation, according to smoking status and randomised treatment regime. Men*

| Cigarettes at entry | Age | Treated | | | | Controls | |
| | | Bendrofluazide | | Propranolol | | Placebo | |
		N	Rate	N	Rate	N	Rate
Smokers:	35–44	3	3.5	3	3.3	4	2.1
	45–54	13	8.7	16	11.2	29	10.0
	55–64	18	16.5	18	17.2	48	23.1
	Total[a]	34	10.1	37	11.4	81	12.6
Non-smokers	35–44	5	3.1	4	2.4	7	2.2
	45–54	15	4.6	11	3.2	35	5.3
	55–64	26	10.1	23	8.6	58	10.8
	Total[a]	46	6.1	38	4.8	100	6.4
	Total[a]	80	7.3	75	6.8	181	8.2

[a] Age-adjusted rates.

Tables 10.3 and 10.4 show all deaths, and all-causes mortality rates in men and women according to their smoking habits at entry to the trial. The data show, as would be expected, consistent differences in overall mortality between smokers and non-smokers in each sex and in each treatment group. In the MRC trial antihypertensive treatment appeared to have no effect on total mortality in either smokers or non-smokers.

Table 10.4. *All deaths and all-causes mortality/1000 person-years of observation, according to smoking status and randomised treatment regime. Women*

| Cigarettes at entry | Age | Treated | | | | Controls | |
| | | Bendrofluazide | | Propranolol | | Placebo | |
		N	Rate	N	Rate	N	Rate
Smokers:	35–44	–	0.0	3	8.1	4	5.1
	45–54	4	3.7	6	5.3	13	5.4
	55–64	9	7.2	8	6.7	21	9.2
	Total[a]	13	4.7	17	6.4	38	7.1
Non-smokers	35–44	2	1.8	–	0.0	1	0.4
	45–54	12	4.0	11	3.5	11	1.9
	55–64	19	5.7	17	5.0	22	3.2
	Total[a]	33	4.4**	28	3.6	34	2.3
	Total[a]	46	4.5	45	4.3	72	3.5

[a] Age-adjusted rates.
Rate significantly different from control group rate **$P < 0.01$.

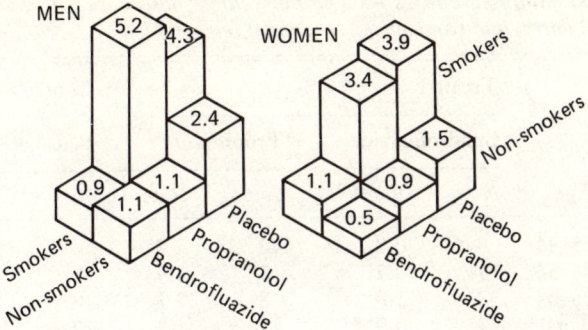

Fig. 10.1. *Stroke incidence per 1000 person-years in men and women according to randomised treatment regimes and cigarette smoking status at entry to the trial.*

The incidence of stroke according to smoking status is shown for the two sexes in Tables 10.5 and 10.6 and diagrammatically in Fig. 10.1. In untreated control subjects and in those randomised to propranolol the stroke rate is 2–3 times greater, and statistically highly significantly greater, in smokers than in non-smokers in the two sexes. In those randomised to bendrofluazide there was little difference in stroke incidence between smokers and non-smokers in either men or women. The overall incidence among smokers in the bendrofluazide group (for both sexes together and all age groups pooled) was 1.0/1000 person-years, a 75% reduction on the rate of 4.0/1000 in controls; bendrofluazide was also associated with a reduction in stroke incidence among non-smokers, from 1.9/1000 to 0.8/1000 (59%). Smokers in the propranolol group, on the other hand, appeared to obtain no stroke benefit (incidence 4.3/1000, an 8% increase) although among non-smokers propranolol seemed also to be associated with a reduced incidence of 1.0/1000 person-years (a 47% reduction) compared with untreated controls.

The clear demonstration in both sexes that the untreated stroke rates in smokers are 2–3 times higher than in non-smokers is obviously important. The trial, however, was not designed to investigate the effect of cigarette smoking on stroke and can provide no evidence that stopping smoking would be beneficial from this point of view; independent data, nevertheless, suggest that the cardiovascular risks of smoking are reversible in those who stop smoking (US Department of Health and Human Services Reports, 1983; Doll, 1983). The MRC trial does suggest that if all mildly hypertensive people were able to answer 'No' to the question 'Do you currently smoke cigarettes?' the stroke incidence would be much lower than it is.

Table 10.5. *Strokes and stroke rates/1000 person-years of observation according to smoking status at entry, and randomised treatment regime. Men*

| | | Treated | | | | Controls | |
| | | Bendrofluazide | | Propranolol | | Placebo | |
Cigarettes at entry	Age	N	Rate	N	Rate	N	Rate
Smokers:	35–44	–	0.0	2	2.2	–	0.0
	45–54	1	0.7	7	4.9	9	3.1
	55–64	2	1.8	8	7.7	18	8.7
	Total[a]	3	0.9**++	17	5.2	27	4.3
Non-smokers	35–44	–	0.0	1	0.6	1	0.3
	45–54	1	0.3	2	0.6	14	2.1
	55–64	7	2.7	6	2.2	22	4.1
	Total[a]	8	1.1	9	1.1	37	2.4
	Total[a]	11	1.0**+	26	2.3	64	2.9

[a] Age-adjusted rates.
Rate significantly different from control group rate **$P < 0.01$.
Rate significantly different from propranolol group rate ++$P < 0.01$, +$P < 0.05$.

Table 10.6. *Strokes and stroke rates/1000 person-years of observation according to smoking status at entry, and randomised treatment regime. Women*

| | | Treated | | | | Controls | |
| | | Bendrofluazide | | Propranolol | | Placebo | |
Cigarettes at entry	Age	N	Rate	N	Rate	N	Rate
Smokers:	35–44	–	0.0	2	5.4	4	5.1
	45–54	1	0.9	2	1.8	8	3.4
	55–64	2	1.6	5	4.2	9	4.0
	Total[a]	3	1.1	9	3.4	21	3.9
Non-smokers	35–44	1	0.9	–	0.0	1	0.4
	45–54	1	0.3	2	0.6	3	0.5
	55–64	2	0.6	6	1.5	19	2.8
	Total[a]	4	0.5	7	0.9	23	1.5
	Total[a]	7	0.7**	16	1.5	44	2.2

[a] Age-adjusted rates.
Rate significantly different from control group rate **$P < 0.01$.

Table 10.7. *All coronary events and rates/1000 person-years of observation according to smoking status and randomised treatment regime. Men*

| Cigarettes at entry | Age | Treated | | | | Controls | |
| | | Bendrofluazide | | Propranolol | | Placebo | |
		N	Rate	N	Rate	N	Rate
Smokers:	35–44	7	8.3	5	5.5	9	4.7
	45–54	19	12.8	22	15.5	36	12.4
	55–64	17	15.6	18	17.2	38	18.3
	Total[a]	43	12.7	45	13.8	83	12.6
Non-smokers	35–44	4	2.5	4	2.4	8	2.5
	45–54	14	4.3	17	5.0	46	7.0
	55–64	38	14.8	18	6.7	62	11.5
	Total[a]	56	7.4	39	5.0*	116	7.5
	Total[a]	99	9.1	84	7.6	199	9.0

[a] Age-adjusted rates.
Rate significantly different from control group rate $*P < 0.05$.

Table 10.8. *All coronary events and rates/1000 person-years of observation according to smoking status and randomised treatment regime. Women*

| Cigarettes at entry | Age | Treated | | | | Controls | |
| | | Bendrofluazide | | Propranolol | | Placebo | |
		N	Rate	N	Rate	N	Rate
Smokers:	35–44	1	2.2	1	2.7	–	0.0
	45–54	5	4.6	4	3.6	8	3.4
	55–64	8	6.4	7	5.9	11	4.8
	Total[a]	14	5.1	12	4.5	19	3.5
Non-smokers	35–44	–	0.0	–	0.0	1	0.4
	45–54	2	0.7	1	0.3	1	0.2
	55–64	4	1.2	5	1.5	13	1.9
	Total[a]	6	0.8	6	0.8	15	1.0
	Total[a]	20	2.0	18	1.7	34	1.7

[a] Age-adjusted rates.

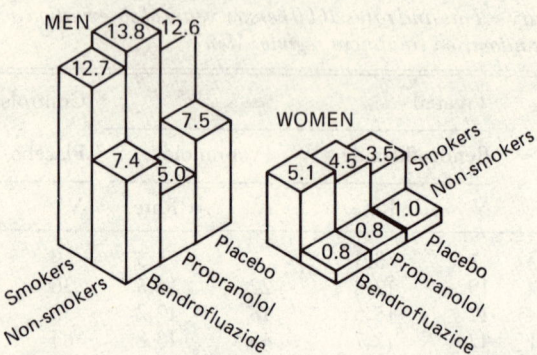

Fig. 10.2. *The incidence of coronary events per 1000 person-years in men and women according to randomised treatment regimes and cigarette smoking status at entry to the trial.*

Coronary events occurred more frequently among smokers than non-smokers in all treatment groups and both sexes (Tables 10.7 and 10.8) and Fig. 10.2. The relative cardiovascular risks for smokers compared with non-smokers were greater for women than they were for men. There was no suggestion that antihypertensive therapy reduced the incidence of coronary events in smokers; indeed the incidence was marginally higher in smokers on either of the two active drugs than in untreated controls. This was true of both sexes. Among non-smokers treated with propranolol the incidence of coronary events was reduced by 33% compared with controls, and by 30% compared with those treated with bendrofluazide, whereas non-smokers treated with bendrofluazide showed virtually the same incidence of CHD events as untreated controls (a 4% reduction).

Tables 10.9 and 10.10 show the incidence of all cardiovascular events in smokers and in non-smokers in men and women respectively. In both sexes the difference in incidence between smokers and non-smokers is greater than the difference in incidence between treated and untreated people. In smokers there is no sign of overall benefit from treatment (Fig. 10.3). In non-smokers both sexes show benefit from active treatment which is largely attributable to the effects of the beta-blocker; indeed, on the basis of once-off conventional chi-squared testing at the end of the trial, the difference in the overall (both sexes/all age groups) incidence of all cardiovascular events between the beta-blocker group and untreated controls was statistically significant ($P < 0.002$).

Blood pressures, after correcting for weight, were slightly higher in smokers than in non-smokers, and especially in the propranolol group tended to increase more after entry to the trial. In the beta-blocker

Table 10.9. *All cardiovascular events and rates/1000 person-years of observation according to smoking status and randomised treatment regime. Men*

| Cigarettes at entry | Age | Treated | | | | Controls | |
| | | Bendrofluazide | | Propranolol | | Placebo | |
		N	Rate	N	Rate	N	Rate
Smokers:	35–44	7	8.3	7	7.7	9	4.7
	45–54	21	14.1	30	21.1	47	16.2
	55–64	20	18.3	26	24.9	60	28.9
	Total[a]	48	14.2	63	19.3	116	17.8
Non-smokers	35–44	4	2.5	5	3.0	9	2.8
	45–54	16	4.9	18	5.3	60	9.1
	55–64	45	17.5	25	9.3	85	15.8
	Total[a]	65	8.6	48	6.1**	154	9.9
	Total[a]	113	10.4	111	10.0	270	12.2

[a] Age-adjusted rates.
Rate significantly different from control group rate **$P < 0.01$.

Table 10.10. *All cardiovascular events and rates/1000 person-years of observation according to smoking status and randomised treatment regime. Women*

| Cigarettes at entry | Age | Treated | | | | Controls | |
| | | Bendrofluazide | | Propranolol | | Placebo | |
		N	Rate	N	Rate	N	Rate
Smokers:	35–44	1	2.2	3	8.1	4	5.1
	45–54	6	5.5	6	5.3	15	5.3
	55–64	10	8.0	12	10.1	22	9.7
	Total[a]	17	6.1	21	7.9	41	7.6
Non-smokers	35–44	1	0.9	–	0.0	2	0.9
	45–54	3	1.0	3	1.0	5	0.9
	55–64	6	1.8	10	2.9	32	4.7
	Total[a]	10	1.3	13	1.7	39	2.6
	Total[a]	27	2.6	34	3.3	80	3.9

[a] Age-adjusted rates.

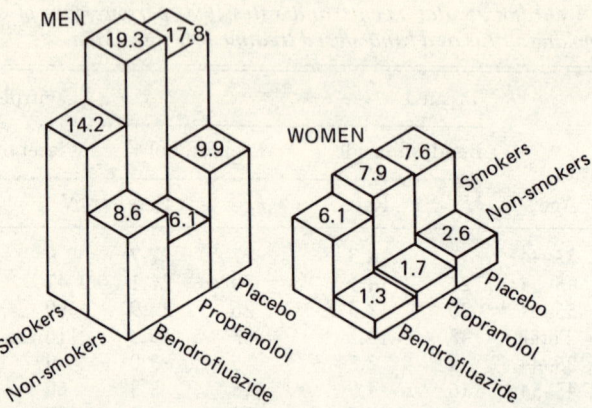

Fig. 10.3. *The incidence of all cardiovascular events per 1000 person-years in men and women according to randomised treatment regimes and cigarette smoking status at entry to the trial.*

group blood pressures were less well controlled in smokers than in non-smokers, as discussed in Chapter 5.

There are pharmacological reasons which may explain why pro-pranolol, a non-selective beta-blocker, might show beneficial results only in non-smokers. Smoking raises plasma adrenalin concentrations and among its short-term effects are increases both in the heart rate and the systolic pressure (Cryer, Haymond, Santiago and Shah, 1976; Trap-Jensen, Carlsen, Lysbo-Svendsen and Christensen, 1979). In the presence of high plasma adrenalin concentrations non-selective beta-blockers can cause a pressor response. This effect is thought to be due to the blocking of beta (1) and beta (2) receptors resulting in unbridled alpha constriction as the pressor response is not seen with cardioselective beta-blockers (Ablad, Carlsson, Johnsson and Regardh, 1980; Struthers, Reid, McLean and Rodger, 1981; Fox, Deanfield, Selwyn, Krikler and Wright, 1983). Bendrofluazide and propranolol are also metabolised differently, bendrofluazide by a mechanism unaffected by smoking but propranolol by smoking-induced hepatic enzymes which enhance its breakdown in the liver. Plasma levels of propranolol have been found to be lower in smokers than in non-smokers (Fox *et al.*, 1983).

The different effects of the thiazide and the beta-blocker in the treatment of mild hypertension among smokers and non-smokers were first recognised at about the time that the sequential analysis had shown treatment to confer benefit in terms of stroke reduction. It was one of the sub-group analyses which looked potentially important but had not been part of the primary analyses planned *ab initio*; interaction between the drugs and cigarette smoking had not been anticipated when the trial was planned, and there was danger in drawing conclusions from sub-group analyses which had only been undertaken in the light of the trial results at that time.

The need to explore the strength of the interaction between smoking and the type of drug taken in determining event rates was clear cut, and multiple logistic regression analyses were undertaken at regular intervals from June 1983 onward to indicate which variables, and which interactions between them, were important from the prognostic point of view.

The values of the variables considered in these analyses were those measured at entry to the trial. The logistic regressions used a controlled step-down procedure, with some categorisation of continuous variables where necessary because of limitations on computer space, The variables considered were:

Age (in six 5-year age groups)
Sex
Cigarette smoking (Yes/No)
Ischaemic ECG changes (Yes/No)
Serum cholesterol level (in two groups >6.5 mmol/l and
    <6.5 mmol/l)
Systolic pressure (in six 10-mm Hg groups)
Diastolic pressure (in five 4-mm Hg groups)
Treatment (placebo/active, as randomised)
Drug regime (propranolol/bendrofluazide, as randomised).

Interactions were tested for each main variable with treatment, drug regime and age.

The results of these logistic regression analyses for the final trial data are shown for all-causes mortality, for stroke, for coronary events, and for all cardiovascular events in Table 10.11.

For all-causes mortality, systolic pressure, increasing age, male sex, cigarette smoking, the presence of ischaemic changes (Minnesota Codes 1_{1-2}, 4_{1-3}, 5_{1-2}) in the ECG, and raised serum cholesterol levels were independently associated with increased mortality.

For stroke, systolic and diastolic pressure, increasing age, male sex, cigarette smoking, treatment status and type of drug were independently associated with stroke incidence, and ischaemic ECG changes approached significance at the 5% level ($P = 0.06$).

For coronary events, systolic pressure, increasing age, male sex, smoking, ischaemic ECG changes, cholesterol level and body mass index all significantly influenced outcome; diastolic pressure, after allowing for the effects of systolic pressure, did not. When the cholesterol data were analysed as a continuum (rather than dichotomised), the change in the relative risk of a coronary event for each

Table 10.11. *The contribution of baseline variables to the risks of developing a trial-terminating event*

	SBP, 10-mm Hg increase	DBP, 4-mm Hg increase	Age, 5-y increase	Female : male	Smokers : non-smokers	Ischaemic ECG : non-ischaemic ECG*	Cholesterol >6.5 : <6.5 mmol/l	Body mass index 3.0 increase	Placebo : active	Propranolol : bendrofluazide
All-causes mortality										
P value	0.03	0.82	<10^{-4}	<10^{-4}	<10^{-4}	<10^{-4}	0.005	0.78	0.86	0.71
RR (95% CL)	1.07	1.01	1.41	0.41	1.99	2.27	1.31	1.01	1.02	0.95
	(1.01–1.14)	(0.94–1.09)	(1.31–1.52)	(0.34–0.50)	(1.66–2.40)	(1.72–3.00)	(1.09–1.58)	(0.93–1.10)	(0.85–1.22)	(0.73–1.23)
Stroke										
P value	0.02	0.003	<10^{-4}	0.002	<10^{-4}	0.06	0.43	0.19	0.0006	0.002
RR (95% CL)	1.14	1.21	1.46	0.60	2.29	1.65	1.14	0.91	1.74	2.30
	(1.02–1.28)	(1.07–1.37)	(1.28–1.66)	(0.43–0.83)	(1.68–3.13)	(1.00–2.69)	(0.83–1.56)	(0.80–1.05)	(1.26–2.40)	(1.33–3.99)
Coronary events										
P value	0.001	0.71	<10^{-4}	<10^{-4}	<10^{-4}	<10^{-4}	<10^{-4}	0.008	0.60	0.24
RR (95% CL)	1.10	1.02	1.32	0.15	2.27	2.13	1.76	1.13	1.05	0.85
	(1.03–1.18)	(0.94–1.10)	(1.23–1.43)	(0.11–0.19)	(1.87–2.76)	(1.56–2.90)	(1.45–2.14)	(1.03–1.23)	(0.87–1.27)	(0.64–1.11)
All cardiovascular events										
P value	0.001	0.05	<10^{-4}	<10^{-4}	<10^{-4}	<10^{-4}	<10^{-4}	0.19	0.01	0.76
RR (95% CL)	1.11	1.07	1.38	0.23	2.36	1.94	1.60	1.05	1.23	1.04
	(1.04–1.17)	(1.00–1.14)	(1.29–1.47)	(0.19–0.28)	(2.01–2.79)	(1.48–2.54)	(1.35–1.89)	(0.98–1.13)	(1.05–1.46)	(0.81–1.32)

* $1_{1-2}4_{1-3}5_{1-2}$ (One or more code present).

mmol/l change in serum cholesterol, was calculated as 1.30 (95% confidence limits 1.17 to 1.45).

Systolic and diastolic pressure, age, sex, smoking status, ECG, cholesterol and randomisation to either active or placebo tablets each predicted the incidence of all cardiovascular events.

When the response to active as opposed to placebo tablets in non-smokers was compared with that in smokers no statistically significant differences were found for all-causes mortality ($P = 0.19$), for stroke ($P = 0.19$), or for coronary events ($P = 0.08$). For all cardiovascular events the difference between smokers and non-smokers was just significant ($P = 0.05$), with the greater benefit in non-smokers.

The interaction between smoking and the response to the two active drugs in determining event rates was more interesting. All-causes mortality was not significantly affected by either drug in smokers or non-smokers, and the drugs were not significantly different ($P = 0.11$) from each other in this respect. The stroke rate was reduced in both smokers and non-smokers on bendrofluazide but was reduced only in non-smokers on propranolol. The difference between the two drugs was significant in this case ($P = 0.03$).

The coronary event rate was not influenced by bendrofluazide in either smokers or non-smokers, and appeared not to be influenced by propranolol in smokers. The rate in non-smokers on propranolol was reduced but the difference between the two drugs in this respect was not statistically significant ($P = 0.11$). A chi-squared test of the difference between the coronary incidence of 2.9 events/1000 person-years in non-smokers in the propranolol group (both sexes and all age groups) and that among non-smoking controls – 4.3 events/1000 person-years – showed significance ($P = 0.03$), at the end of the trial.

The rate for all cardiovascular events was also not influenced by bendrofluazide in either smokers or non-smokers, neither was it affected by propranolol in smokers. In non-smokers the rate was reduced and the difference between the two drugs in this respect was significant ($P = 0.01$). A one-off chi-squared test at the end of the trial showed the difference between the rate for all cardiovascular events in non-smokers on propranolol (both sexes and all age groups) – 3.9/1000 person-years – and that in non-smoking controls – 6.3/1000 person-years (a 38% reduction with the drug) – to be significant ($P = 0.002$).

Clearly these interesting relationships between the effectiveness of the beta-blockers and smoking status would need independent confirmation. If that were forthcoming they might provide the first real evidence of an effective pharmacological measure for the *primary* prevention of coronary disease.

11 ECG abnormalities as predictors of morbidity and mortality in treated and untreated mild hypertension

Changes in the incidence of electrocardiographic abnormalities which appeared to be drug related were described in Chapter 7. They included differences in the incidence rates of ECG evidence of possible transmural myocardial infarction between those treated with the thiazide and the beta-blocker; the thiazide group showed a significant excess compared with untreated controls whereas the propranolol group showed a significantly reduced incidence of such changes compared with controls.

Propranolol was more effective in preventing the development of left axis deviation than was bendrofluazide, but bendrofluazide appeared to be markedly more effective than propranolol in preventing the amplitude changes of left ventricular hypertrophy. The two drugs had different effects on cardiac repolarisation in the two sexes. In women bendrofluazide was associated with a significantly higher incidence of ST depression and of T-wave abnormalities alone than in control women. These changes were largely attributable to hypokalaemia. No comparable effects were found in men; indeed the incidence of T-wave changes alone was significantly reduced in men on bendrofluazide. Propranolol, on the other hand, was associated with lower rates of ST depression in men and with higher rates of T-wave inversion in women. Reduced rates of both atrial and ventricular ectopic arrhythmias were associated with propranolol treatment. At an earlier stage of the trial (and also in a specially mounted sub-study), increased rates of ventricular ectopic arrhythmias in those on thiazide had been found.

In this chapter the relationships between ECG changes and morbidity and mortality are examined according to the treatment regime to which people had been allocated. As a result of the exclusion factors operating before a person was accepted into the trial, there were few with severely abnormal ECGs at the entry examination. The relationship between ECG abnormalities and outcome was investigated by determining the incidence of trial-terminating events according to the

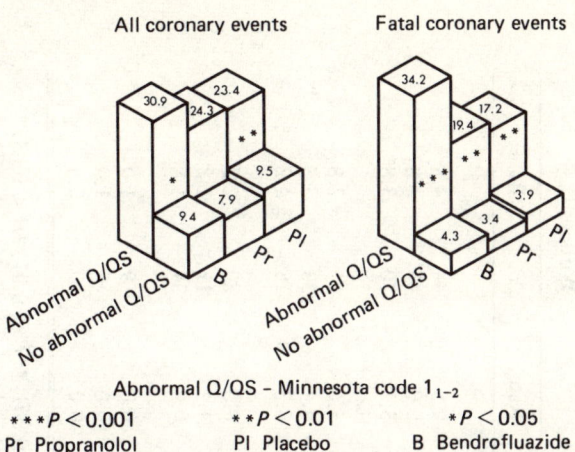

Fig. 11.1. *The incidence per 1000 person-years of all coronary events and of fatal coronary events in men with and without ECG changes compatible with myocardial infarction, according to randomised treatment regime. (The asterisks indicate the significance of differences in event rates between those with and without the ECG abnormality, and apply to Figs. 11.1 to 11.6).*

latest (pre-event) reading for each individual. Many of the abnormalities would have developed during the course of the study and some of them, as described above, would have been induced by the drugs themselves. The numbers of events, when broken down by ECG category, were sometimes too small for reliable significance testing; the small number of cardiovascular events in women, in particular, frequently prevented useful analyses.

ECG abnormalities as predictors of cardiovascular complications

The prognostic significance of abnormal Q/QS items (Minnesota Code 1_{1-2}) in terms of all-causes mortality, all cardiovascular events, all coronary events, and fatal coronary events is shown for the two sexes in Table 11.1. The coronary data are illustrated for men only in Fig. 11.1. These more definite changes of possible myocardial infarction were associated with increased all-causes mortality which was greater, but not significantly greater, for those on active therapy. A similar pattern was present for all cardiovascular terminating events. For all coronary events, and for fatal coronary events, the excess of events was greater in the thiazide group but the numbers were too small for the differences to be significant. Clearly abnormal Q/QS items in men had considerable prognostic significance, but the data for women were insufficient to be certain.

Table 11.1. *The predictive value for various categories of trial-terminating events, of ECG evidence of transmural infarction abnormal Q/QS (Minnesota Code 1$_{1-2}$), in men and women, according to randomised treatment regime*

	Men				Women			
	With 1$_{1-2}$		Without 1$_{1-2}$		With 1$_{1-2}$		Without 1$_{1-2}$	
	N	Rate	N	Rate	N	Rate	N	Rate
All-causes mortality								
Bendrofluazide	9	37.4***	73	7.4	2	9.5	44	4.8
Propranolol	7	34.0**	68	6.7	–	0.0	45	4.8
Placebo	12	22.4*	169	8.5	2	5.3	70	3.8
All cardiovascular events								
Bendrofluazide	8	34.2**	105	10.7	1	5.6	26	2.8
Propranolol	7	34.1*	105	10.3	1	4.4	33	3.5
Placebo	14	30.8***	257	12.9	2	5.3	78	4.2
All coronary events								
Bendrofluazide	7	30.9*	92	9.4	–	0.0	20	2.2
Propranolol	5	24.3	80	7.9	1	4.4	17	1.8
Placebo	10	23.4**	190	9.5	–	0.0	34	1.8
Fatal coronary events								
Bendrofluazide	8	34.2***	42	4.3	–	0.0	9	1.0
Propranolol	4	19.4**	34	3.4	–	0.0	5	1.0
Placebo	9	17.2**	78	3.9	–	0.0	10	0.5

Rate differs significantly from the rate in those without ECG abnormality, *** $P < 0.001$, ** $P < 0.01$, * $P < 0.05$. In Tables 11.1 to 11.5 N indicates the number of subjects with, or without, the ECG abnormality who had terminating events.

Table 11.2. *The predictive value for various categories of trial-terminating events, of left axis deviation (Minnesota Code 2_1), by sex and treatment regime*

	Men				Women			
	With 2_1		Without 2_1		With 2_1		Without 2_1	
	N	Rate	N	Rate	N	Rate	N	Rate
All-causes mortality								
Bendrofluazide	5	6.8	77	8.2	6	12.6*	40	4.5
Propranolol	5	7.1	70	7.2	3	8.3	42	4.6
Placebo	17	12.5	164	8.7	3	4.0	69	3.8
All cardiovascular events								
Bendrofluazide	8	11.0	105	11.2	3	5.2	24	2.7
Propranolol	5	15.2	107	11.0	4	10.0	30	3.3
Placebo	25	17.1	246	13.0	6	6.3	74	4.1
All coronary events								
Bendrofluazide	8	11.0	91	9.7	2	3.7	18	2.0
Propranolol	2	7.0	83	8.5	2	6.6	16	1.8
Placebo	16	11.6	184	9.7	2	1.5	32	1.8
Fatal coronary events								
Bendrofluazide	5	6.8	45	4.8	1	2.2	8	0.9
Propranolol	1	1.3	37	3.8	1	5.0	8	0.9
Placebo	8	5.3	79	4.2	–	0.0	10	0.6

Rate differs significantly from the rate in those without ECG abnormality, *$P < 0.05$.

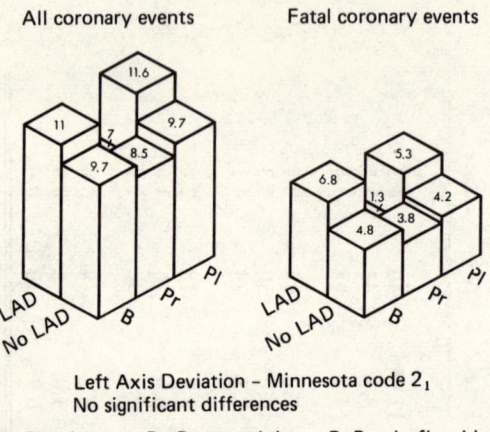

All coronary events   Fatal coronary events

Left Axis Deviation – Minnesota code 2_1
No significant differences

Pl Placebo   Pr Propranolol   B Bendrofluazide

Fig. 11.2. *The incidence per 1000 person-years of all coronary events and of fatal coronary events in men with and without left-axis deviation, according to random-ised treatment regime.*

Among men with the most certain changes of infarction in their final electrocardiograms (Minnesota Code 1_1), there were 6 deaths (5 recorded as due to coronary heart disease) among the 43 person-years of men being treated with bendrofluazide (giving an age-adjusted rate of 141 per 1000 person-years), 3 deaths among the 36 person-years of such men being treated with propranolol (78 per 1000 person years), and 5 deaths in 127 person-years of observation in such men on placebo (33 per 1000 person-years). Only in this small group of men with the strongest ECG evidence of infarction was the mortality significantly increased in the bendrofluazide group, compared with controls ($P = 0.03$).

Left axis deviation appeared to be unrelated to prognosis in the trial. This was true for both sexes and for both treated and control subjects (Table 11.2 and Fig. 11.2). The presence of tall R waves in left ventricular leads (Minnesota Code 3_1), which is an early manifestation of LVH in some subjects, appeared to be of some prognostic value for all cardiovascular events but only in untreated subjects (Table 11.3 and Fig. 11.3). The curiously high rate of deaths from all-causes in women whose tall R waves persisted despite thiazide treatment was not matched by a similar trend in men and remains unexplained. Perhaps it was a chance finding.

The presence of ST segment depression and T-wave inversion or flattening (4_{1-3} with 5_{1-3}) was significantly associated with increased mortality and cardiovascular morbidity in both the control subjects

Table 11.3. *The predictive value for various categories of trial-terminating events, of left ventricular hypertrophy (Minnesota Code 3_1), by sex and treatment regime*

	Men				Women			
	With 3_1		Without 3_1		With 3_1		Without 3_1	
	N	Rate	N	Rate	N	Rate	N	Rate
All-causes mortality								
Bendrofluazide	3	5.6	79	8.2	7	22.1**	39	4.3
Propranolol	4	6.0	71	7.3	4	10.1	41	4.5
Placebo	17	12.6	164	8.6	4	2.9	68	3.8
All cardiovascular events								
Bendrofluazide	6	12.3	107	11.2	1	2.8	26	2.9
Propranolol	6	11.5	106	10.9	2	4.6	32	3.5
Placebo	27	19.9	244	12.8	5	3.6	75	4.2
All coronary events								
Bendrofluazide	5	10.4	94	9.8	1	2.8	19	2.1
Propranolol	4	7.8	81	8.3	2	4.6	16	1.8
Placebo	16	11.9	184	9.7	1	0.7	33	1.9
Fatal coronary events								
Bendrofluazide	1	1.9	49	5.1	1	2.8	8	0.9
Propranolol	2	3.4	36	3.7	1	2.7	8	0.9
Placebo	8	5.8	79	4.2	1	0.7	–	0.5

Rate differs significantly from the rate in those without ECG abnormality, *** $P < 0.001$, ** $P < 0.01$, * $P < 0.05$.

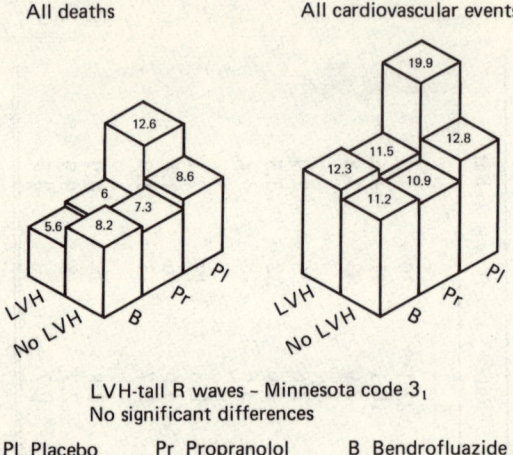

LVH-tall R waves – Minnesota code 3_1
No significant differences

Pl Placebo   Pr Propranolol   B Bendrofluazide

Fig. 11.3. *The incidence per 1000 person-years of all deaths and of all cardio-vascular events in men with and without left ventricular hypertrophy, according to randomised treatment regime.*

and in those on propranolol (Table 11.4 and Fig. 11.4). It was clearly of less prognostic value in those treated with the thiazide. The highly significantly increased incidence of such ECG changes in women treated with the thiazide has been described in Chapter 7; in men the incidence of such changes did not appear to be induced by thiazide treatment. But in both sexes repolarisation abnormalities in those on treatment with bendrofluazide did not appear to have the same medical significance as similar changes occurring in the other two treatment groups.

For women, among whom the thiazide induced a high incidence of T-wave inversion and flattening (5_{1-3}), there was no suggestion that this type of abnormality was associated with increased morbidity; in men, among whom the thiazide reduced the incidence of T-wave changes, the abnormality was associated with significantly higher event rates than occurred in men without them. The data are shown in Table 11.5 and illustrated in Fig. 11.5.

The number of subjects with codable ventricular ectopic arrhythmias was not large. There were 78 person-years of observation for men with this abnormality in the thiazide group, 49 person-years for men in the propranolol group and 143 for men on placebo. Coronary deaths numbered 5, 0 and 4 in the three groups, respectively. The age adjusted coronary mortality rates are illustrated in Fig. 11.6. These data concerning cardiac arrhythmias, are based on very small numbers. Supraventricular ectopic beats were not associated with excess morbidity.

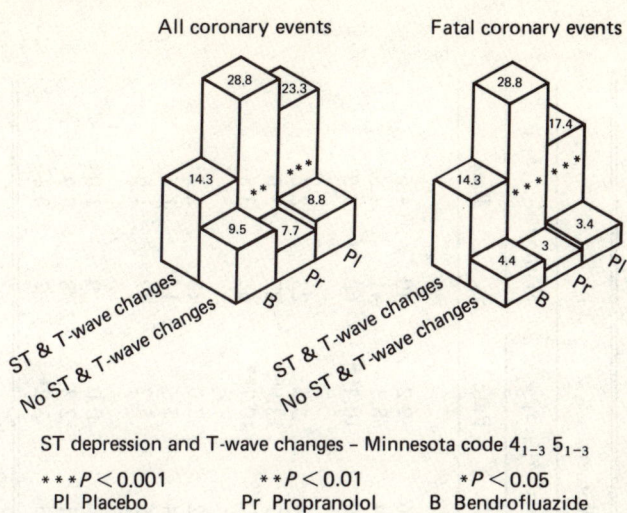

All coronary events   Fatal coronary events

ST depression and T-wave changes – Minnesota code 4_{1-3} 5_{1-3}

* * * $P < 0.001$ * * $P < 0.01$ * $P < 0.05$
Pl Placebo   Pr Propranolol   B Bendrofluazide

Fig. 11.4. *The incidence per 1000 person-years of all coronary events and of fatal coronary events in men with and without ST segment depression and T-wave changes, according to randomised treatment regime.*

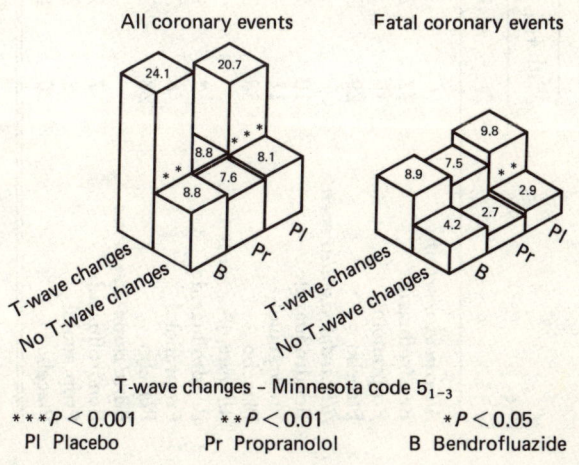

All coronary events   Fatal coronary events

T-wave changes – Minnesota code 5_{1-3}

* * * $P < 0.001$ * * $P < 0.01$ * $P < 0.05$
Pl Placebo   Pr Propranolol   B Bendrofluazide

Fig. 11.5. *The incidence per 1000 person-years of all coronary events and of fatal coronary events in men with and without T-wave changes, according to randomised treatment regime.*

Table 11.4. *The predictive value for various categories of trial-terminating events of repolarisation abnormalities – ST depression with T-wave changes – (Minnesota Code 4_{1-3}, 5_{1-3}) by sex and treatment regime*

	Men				Women			
	With 4_{1-3}, 5_{1-3}		Without 4_{1-3}, 5_{1-3}		With 4_{1-3}, 5_{1-3}		Without 4_{1-3}, 5_{1-3}	
	N	Rate	N	Rate	N	Rate	N	Rate
All-causes mortality								
Bendrofluazide	12	23.4*	70	7.2	6	9.2	40	4.6
Propranolol	10	35.6***	65	6.5	4	8.1	41	4.5
Placebo	29	26.6***	152	7.8	10	10.4**	62	3.5
All cardiovascular events								
Bendrofluazide	10	13.2	103	10.7	4	5.8	23	2.6
Propranolol	11	45.0***	101	10.1	7	13.9***	27	3.0
Placebo	38	31.6***	233	12.0	12	10.7***	68	3.8
All coronary events								
Bendrofluazide	7	14.4	92	9.5	2	3.0	18	2.1
Propranolol	8	28.9**	77	7.7	4	7.5	14	1.5
Placebo	28	23.3***	172	8.8	5	5.2	29	1.6
Fatal coronary events								
Bendrofluazide	7	14.3	43	4.4	–	0.0	9	1.0
Propranolol	8	28.8***	30	3.0	1	2.3	8	0.9
Placebo	20	17.4***	67	3.4	3	3.2*	7	0.4

Rate differs significantly from the rate in those without ECG abnormality, *** $P < 0.001$, ** $P < 0.01$, * $P < 0.05$.

Table 11.5. *The predictive value for various categories of trial-terminating events, of repolarisation abnormalities – T-wave changes in the absence of ST depression – (Minnesota Code 5_{1-3} alone) by sex and treatment regime*

	Men				Women			
	With 5_{1-3}		Without 5_{1-3}		With 5_{1-3}		Without 5_{1-3}	
	N	Rate	N	Rate	N	Rate	N	Rate
All-causes mortality								
Bendrofluazide	9	18.5*	61	6.6	4	6.6	36	4.4
Propranolol	9	14.8*	56	5.9	4	7.1	37	4.4
Placebo	19	15.4**	133	7.3	7	6.3	55	3.2
All cardiovascular events								
Bendrofluazide	11	24.1*	92	10.0	1	1.6	22	2.7
Propranolol	9	14.1	92	9.7	3	4.9	24	2.8
Placebo	35	29.5***	198	10.8	5	4.6	63	3.7
All coronary events								
Bendrofluazide	11	24.1**	81	8.8	1	1.6	17	2.1
Propranolol	5	8.8	72	7.6	3	4.9	11	1.3
Placebo	24	20.7***	148	8.1	1	0.9	28	1.7
Fatal coronary events								
Bendrofluazide	4	8.9	39	4.2	–	0.0	9	1.1
Propranolol	4	7.5	26	2.7	1	2.2	7	0.8
Placebo	13	9.8**	54	2.9	–	0.0	7	0.4

Rate differs significantly from the rate in those without ECG abnormality, ***$P < 0.001$, **$P < 0.01$, *$P < 0.05$.

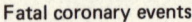

Fatal coronary events

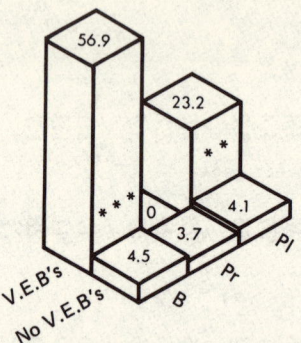

Ventricular ectopic arrhythmia – Minnesota code 8₁ (v)

***$P < 0.001$ **$P < 0.01$ *$P < 0.05$
Pl Placebo   Pr Propranolol   B Bendrofluazide

Fig. 11.6. *The incidence per 1000 person-years of fatal coronary events in men with and without ventricular ectopic arrhythmias, according to randomised treatment regime.*

ECG abnormalities as predictors of severe hypertension

Withdrawal from randomised treatment as a result of the development of hypertension of a severity requiring transfer to alternative treatment was unusual for those who had been randomly allocated to groups receiving active drugs. It occurred in only 76 people, 19 in the thiazide group and 57 in the beta-blocker group. Analysis of the rates of withdrawal according to ECG abnormalities left the cells too small to allow useful comparisons within the actively treated groups. Among control subjects, however, 1029 required to be transferred from placebo to active tablets on account of rising blood pressure and this gave adequate numbers for analysis.

Only two ECG abnormalities appeared to predict the development of severe hypertension. Among control subjects with the amplitude criteria for LVH (Minnesota Code 3₁), the rate of withdrawal on blood pressure grounds was higher than among controls without this abnormality, and this was true of both sexes (Table 11.6). In men the rates were 66 and 37 per 1000 person-years respectively; in women they were 38 and 25 per 100 person-years respectively. However, as ECG changes of LVH are found more frequently in those whose blood pressures are towards the top of the trial range, the findings may not mean that LVH in the ECG is indicating patients whose *rate* of rise of pressure is increased.

Table 11.6. *The predictive value for the development of severe hypertension of tall R waves in left ventricular leads, in control men and women*

		With tall R waves in early ECG		Without tall R waves in early ECG	
		N	Rate	N	Rate
Men:	35–44	13	69.5	132	37.4
	45–54	24	64.3	232	35.2
	55–64	21	64.8	189	37.6
	Total	58	65.7	553	36.6
Women:	35–44	6	78.3	66	31.3
	45–54	8	38.1	156	25.4
	55–64	11	25.1	149	22.8
	Total	25	38.2	371	25.1

ECG changes of left ventricular hypertrophy and strain (Minnesota Code 3_1 with 4_{1-3}, 5_{1-2}), also predicted high rates of development of severe levels of hypertension (54/1000 person-years in men, 38/1000 person-years in women compared with 38/1000 and 26/1000 person-years respectively in those without LVH and strain.

Abnormal Q/QS items, left axis deviation, and T-wave inversion did not characterise people at increased risk of developing severe hypertension, and ST segment depression with T-wave inversion appeared valuable as a predictor only in men where those with and without the abnormality had rates of 94.3 and 37.0/1000 person-years respectively. In women the comparable rates were 33.2 and 25.1/1000 person-years.

In general the relationship between ECG abnormalities and cardio-vascular events was as would be expected; those with the abnormality were at greater risk than those without the abnormality in each treatment group. But there were exceptions. Left axis deviation did not predict risk in any group; the amplitude changes of LVH pre-dicted risk in control but not in treated subjects, and the ST segment and T-wave abnormalities apparently induced by the thiazide were not associated with the adverse prognostic significance seen in the propranolol and placebo groups.

Abnormal Q/QS items appeared to be associated with higher all-causes mortality than was present in those without the abnormal-ity. The risk ratio of those with and those without the abnormality was greater in the groups on active treatment. Increased total coronary event rates and increased fatal coronary event rates were present in those with abnormal Q/QS items and this was particularly true of the thiazide group. The numbers involved however were small. For the few with the most definite evidence of infarction (Minnesota Code 1_1), and for those with ventricular ectopic arrhythmias, thiazide treatment did seem to be accompanied by high coronary mortality.

Some rather weak evidence from other major randomised controlled trials, discussed in Chapter 13, has been used to suggest that there may be an increase in risk and particularly in coronary risk, in people on treatment with a thiazide diuretic if they are already showing some evidence of cardiac involvement. In none of the trials, including the MRC trial, is the evidence conclusive. The electrocardiographic evidence reviewed here and in Chapter 7 is, not surprisingly, in general accord with the overall morbidity and mortality data described in Chapter 9. However, there are unexplained discrepancies with regard to the similar incidence of ECG evidence of transmural infarction in the two sexes, and in smokers and non-smokers, and their marked differences in coronary heart attacks.

12 Biochemical characteristics, their changes due to antihypertensive treatment, and their prognostic value

Biochemical investigations were included in the trial protocol for three reasons. At entry it was important to exclude from the trial those whose hypertension was secondary to some remediable condition; during the course of the follow-up the clinics needed to monitor electrolytic and other changes induced by the drugs; and at the conclusion of the study it would be important to see whether groups of people at different risks and with different responses to treatment could be identified and it was hoped that biochemical factors might be useful in specifying their characteristics.

By having all the blood investigations carried out at one central laboratory – the Wolfson Research Laboratories in Birmingham – the problems of inter-laboratory differences in methods and standards were avoided and data of high quality were obtained. The facilities provided for the clinics – centrifuges for those practices which did not already have them, specially designed postal packs, and business reply postal arrangements – are described in Chapter 2. Results of the tests were communicated on cards or as computer print-out to the co-ordinating centre, transferred to the Northwick Park computer and sent to the clinics (with the computer's comments on any action needed) within a few days of a specimen being taken. The procedures worked smoothly and satisfactorily. When the laboratory found abnormal results requiring urgent notification to the patient's doctor this was done by telephone through the co-ordinating centre.

Serum specimens were centrifuged and separated in the clinic and sent by post to the laboratory in Birmingham, where they were usually analysed within 48 h of collection. This procedure worked well, and there were rarely any problems with faulty specimens. A 12-test biochemical profile was measured on each specimen with the Technicon SMA-12 analyser. This was probably the largest and longest attempt at biochemical monitoring of a population group, and some of the lessons learnt are discussed elsewhere (Broughton, Holder and

Ashby, 1986). This Chapter deals with the 6 tests of most direct interest to the trial, namely serum potassium, sodium, urate, urea, cholesterol and glucose.

Few people who passed through the screening and reached the entry examination were then excluded from the trial solely on the grounds of abnormal biochemical findings. We cannot state precisely the proportion of mild hypertensives who were excluded for metabolic reasons. Diabetics, for example, would usually have been detected as a result of urine tests at the time of the entry examination and biochemical confirmation may have been arranged with local laboratories. People found at the entry examination to have a biochemical abnormality, such as a low serum potassium level, for example, would have been referred for the necessary investigations to exclude primary aldosteronism, but the co-ordinating centre did not know the proportion of such cases. Certainly the only case of phaeo-chromocytoma known to have been detected during the trial's screening procedures was found without help from the co-ordinating centre or the laboratory in Birmingham.

Table 12.1 shows the means and standard deviations of serum

Table 12.1. *Mean (M) and s.d. values of serum biochemical characteristics at entry to the*

| | | Men | | | | | |
| | | Bendrofluazide | | Propranolol | | Placebo | |
		Entry	3 y	Entry	3 y	Entry	3 y
Serum potassium (mmol/l)	M	4.11	3.72***	4.11	4.22***	4.13	4.17
	S.D.	0.37	0.51	0.35	0.43	0.37	0.39
Serum sodium (mmol/l)	M	141.6	140.9***	141.6	141.5	141.7	141.6
	S.D.	2.2	2.5	2.2	2.3	2.2	2.3
Serum uric acid (μmol/l)	M	382.3	432.0***	373.7	393.5***	372.6	380.8
	S.D.	70.3	78.6	68.6	68.6	64.5	68.3
Serum urea (mmol/l)	M	5.43	5.98***	5.44	5.76*	5.40	5.63
	S.D.	1.19	1.36	1.18	1.35	1.19	1.37
Serum cholesterol (mmol/l)	M	6.26	6.36***	6.23	6.31**	6.24	6.25
	S.D.	1.01	1.03	1.06	10.8	0.99	0.99
Serum glucose (mmol/l)	M	5.48	5.69*	5.48	5.50*	5.46	5.58
	S.D.	1.04	1.36	1.03	1.18	1.02	1.20

Values refer to difference between changes of levels in treatment group compared with placebo group: ***$P < 0.001$, **$P < 0.01$, *$P < 0.05$.

potassium, sodium, urate, urea, cholesterol and (casual) glucose levels at entry to the trial, and at the annual examination carried out 3 years later. The significances of the differences between the changes in the treated groups and the changes in the control group are also shown.

As expected, the mean serum potassium level fell in the bendrofluazide groups – by 0.39 mmol/l in men and by 0.42 mmol/l in women – changes which were very highly significantly different from those in the placebo group. Those on propranolol, on the other hand, showed increases in serum potassium, in both sexes, of 0.11 mmol/l, which also differed significantly from the changes in the control groups. During the trial 10 men and 17 women were withdrawn from their randomised bendrofluazide on grounds of severe hypokalaemia (serum K <2.5 mmol/l) although it had caused no known morbidity or mortality.

Mean serum sodium levels of both men and women treated with bendrofluazide fell during the 3-year period. The falls were small but were significantly greater than in the control groups.

Serum urate levels showed the greatest increases in subjects on the

trial and at the third annual examination, by sex and randomised treatment regime

		Women					
		Bendrofluazide		Propranolol		Placebo	
		Entry	3 y	Entry	3 y	Entry	3 y
Serum potassium (mmol/l)	M	4.04	3.62***	4.07	4.18***	4.07	4.12
	S.D.	0.39	0.51	0.39	0.45	0.39	0.40
Serum sodium (mmol/l)	M	141.7	141.0***	141.8	141.5*	141.8	141.6
	S.D.	2.2	2.4	2.1	2.4	2.2	2.1
Serum uric acid (μmol/l)	M	298.9	354.6***	292.0	323.0***	293.2	308.3
	S.D.	65.6	75.6	61.0	67.6	60.6	65.6
Serum urea (mmol/l)	M	5.17	5.71***	5.14	5.52***	5.16	5.39
	S.D.	1.21	1.41	1.20	1.29	1.16	1.24
Serum cholesterol (mmol/l)	M	6.67	6.81***	6.67	6.73	6.66	6.71
	S.D.	1.20	1.21	1.15	1.20	1.14	1.16
Serum glucose (mmol/l)	M	5.37	5.50*	5.39	5.39	5.38	5.43
	S.D.	0.92	1.09	0.99	1.00	0.93	1.09

thiazide with smaller increases in those on propranolol; both increases were significantly greater than among controls. Urate levels were higher in men than in women in the trial, and the incidence of gout was consistently higher in men in all treatment groups. Serum urea levels also showed greater increases in treated than in control subjects, especially in those receiving bendrofluazide.

Serum cholesterol level showed a small but statistically significant increase in both men and women on bendrofluazide and a small increase in men on propranolol.

Although impaired glucose metabolism was one of the commoner causes of withdrawal from randomised treatment for both men and women in the thiazide group, the mean changes in serum glucose level occurring in the 3-year interval among those who had not been withdrawn were only marginally higher in the bendrofluazide group than among controls.

The incidence of impaired glucose tolerance was higher in men than in women in each treatment group, as was the 3-year change in serum glucose level. In about 60% of those whose impairment of glucose metabolism had been induced by bendrofluazide, the metabolic abnormality reverted to normal within the year following withdrawal of the drug.

Biochemical factors and their value in the prediction of individual risk

Multiple regression analysis was used to estimate the relation between biochemical characteristics in the serum and the probability of a subsequent terminating event.

The serum biochemical characteristics at entry to the trial which were associated significantly with increased incidence of terminating events (Table 12.2) were: a high cholesterol level (for coronary and

Table 12.2. *The significance of the regression coefficients of biochemical characteristics (in serum at entry to the trial) in predicting subsequent terminating events*

Serum constituent	All causes mortality (P)	Stroke (P)	All cardiovascular events (P)	All coronary events (P)
Potassium	$<10^{-4}$	NS	NS	0.027
Sodium	0.001	NS	0.0007	$<10^{-4}$
Uric acid	NS	NS	NS	NS
Urea	NS	NS	NS	NS
Cholesterol	NS	NS	$<10^{-4}$	$<10^{-4}$
Glucose	NS	NS	NS	NS

NS Not significant.

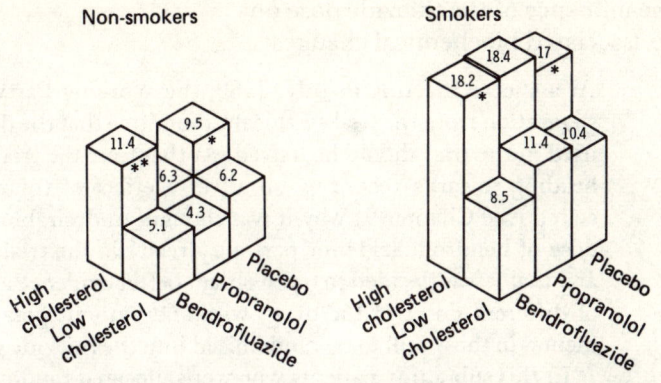

Non-smokers   Smokers

**P < 0.01 | for differences between high cholesterol and low cholesterol group rates
*P < 0.05 |

Fig. 12.1. *The incidence per 1000 person-years of all coronary events in men, according to randomised treatment regime, cigarette smoking status and serum cholesterol level at entry to the trial. (High cholesterol ≥6.5 mmol/l; low cholesterol <6.5 mmol/l.)*

for all cardiovascular events); a below-average serum sodium (for all coronary events, all cardiovascular events and all-causes mortality); a high serum potassium (for coronary events and all-causes mortality). None of these biochemical parameters at entry was significantly correlated with stroke incidence.

The serum cholesterol level was much the most powerful predictor of cardiovascular complications among the biochemical factors measured at entry to the trial, and it was of most predictive value for coronary events (Table 12.2). A 1 mmol/l difference in serum cholesterol was associated with a 1.30 difference in the relative risk of suffering a coronary event.

In the multiple regression analyses, the serum cholesterol was less powerful as a predictor of coronary events, or of all cardiovascular events, than were sex, age, smoking history or evidence of myocardial ischaemia in the latest ECG.

Figure 12.1 illustrates the relationship between entry cholesterol (above or below 6.5 mmol/l) and coronary incidence according to smoking habit at entry to the trial. It would appear that a high cholesterol level and smoking are additive risk factors for coronary heart disease. The figure also suggests that propranolol, like bendrofluazide, is of no value in the prevention of CHD in smokers, whatever the cholesterol level, but that in non-smokers it may be effective even in the presence of hypercholesterolaemia.

Coronary events in women were not sufficiently numerous to allow a similar analysis to be made for them.

The influence of the thiazide dose on the associated biochemical changes

At a special meeting in July, 1980, the Working Party considered a suggestion from the trial's Ethical Committee that the dose of thiazide used in the trial should be halved. At that time the trial seemed to be heading towards recording an adverse effect of thiazide. We have stated (see Chapter 9) why it was thought undesirable to change the dose of bendrofluazide for persons already in the trial on that drug, and that it was decided to try to obtain better evidence about the value of different doses of the drug, with and without potassium supplements, in those still to be randomised into the thiazide group.

In this sub-study patients who were allocated randomly to join the thiazide group were immediately further randomised to one of four groups as follows:

A. 123 people received bendrofluazide 5 mg daily.
B. 113 people received bendrofluazide 10 mg daily, as in the main part of the trial.
C. 123 people received bendrofluazide 5 mg daily plus 16.8 mmol potassium daily.
D. 125 people received bendrofluazide 10 mg daily plus 33.6 mmol potassium daily.

The aim of the study was to compare blood pressure control in the 4 groups and to relate this to subjective adverse reactions and to biochemical changes. The sample size was planned to give a power of 95% for the detection of a 3-mm difference in mean diastolic pressure at 6 months, significant at the 5% level (MRC Working Party, 1986a).

Table 12.3 summarises the results for both sexes pooled. The higher dose of bendrofluazide did not produce a greater reduction in blood pressure. The fall in serum potassium during the first 3 months of the study was dose related ($P = 0.0004$). The reported incidence of subjective adverse reactions, such as lethargy, dizziness, and headache was also dose related ($P = 0.04$). The incidence of symptomatic adverse reactions on the lower dose of thiazide (21.1/ 1000 person-years) was only half that of the high diuretic dose (42.2/1000 person-years). The symptom rate from the placebo group in the trial was about 7/1000 person-years. Unfortunately the numbers were insufficient to be able to show the frequency of specific adverse reactions in relation to thiazide dose, for comparison with the rates of such symptoms in untreated controls.

The increase in serum urea concentration was greater on the higher dose, but the difference was not statistically significant. Serum urate, glucose, cholesterol, and sodium levels showed no evidence of a dose/response effect. Although potassium supplementation appeared to reduce the fall in serum potassium the effect was not statistically

Table 12.3. *The effects of different bendrofluazide doses, with and without potassium supplementation, on blood pressure levels, on serum biochemical values and on subjective adverse reactions. Both sexes together*

	A + C bendrofluazide 5 mg daily (N = 246)		B + D bendrofluazide 10 mg daily (N = 238)		A + B no potassium supplement (N = 236)		C + D potassium supplement (N = 248)	
	Mean	S.D.	Mean	S.D.	Mean	S.D.	Mean	S.D.
Entry blood pressure (mm Hg)								
SBP	160.9	16.6	161.2	15.8	160.5	15.7	161.6	16.7
DBP	98.4	5.9	98.4	5.7	97.8	5.5	99.0	6.0
SBP fall, entry–6 months	27.1	15.7	27.8	15.7	27.0	15.9	27.8	15.5
DBP fall, entry–6 months	13.4	8.7	13.1	8.7	12.9	8.8	13.6	8.6
Entry serum potassium (mmol/l)	4.11	0.37	4.12	0.39	4.08	0.35	4.15	0.41
Potassium fall, entry to 3 months (mmol/l)	0.23***	0.51	0.41	0.45	0.35	0.51	0.29	0.47
Entry serum urea (mmol/l)	5.38	1.28	5.19	1.12	5.23	1.27	5.35	1.15
Serum urea rise, entry–1 y (mmol/l)	0.41	1.25	0.56	1.09	0.55	1.22	0.42	1.13
Entry serum urate (μmol/l)	342.3	82.7	348.4	82.6	339.8	81.1	350.6	84.0
Serum urate rise, entry–1 y (μmol/1)	50.4	59.0	49.9	60.2	54.7	64.6	45.6	53.7
	N	rate[a]	N	rate[a]	N	rate[a]	N	rate[a]
Impaired glucose tolerance	1	1.3	3	4.5	3	4.3	1	1.4
Gout	1	1.3	3	4.5	1	1.4	3	4.2
Subjective adverse reactions	16	21.1*	28	42.2	20	28.4	24	33.5

* $P < 0.05$ for A + C compared with B + D.

*** $P < 0.001$ for A + C compared with B + D.

[a] rate per 1000 patient-years.

significant; likewise the study produced no evidence that the thiazide
supplemented by potassium had a greater effect in lowering blood
pressure than the thiazide alone.

This sub-study confirmed earlier reports showing that increasing
the dose of thiazide above the levels widely accepted as the lower end
of the therapeutic range is unlikely to reduce blood pressure further
and may have adverse effects on serum potassium levels and increase
subjective adverse reactions.

13 Controlled clinical trials in mild hypertension

There had been only two published accounts of the results of controlled trials of the treatment of hypertension at the time the MRC trial was being planned. They were the paper by Hamilton, Thompson and Wisniewski (1964) and the first report of the trial conducted by the US Veterans Administration (Veterans Administration Co-operative Study Group, 1967). Hamilton's study dealt with moderately severe but uncomplicated patients with diastolic (IV) pressures above 110 mm Hg; the first report from the VA trial concerned men with diastolic (V) pressures in the 115 to 129 mm Hg range. Both of these trials reported benefit from treatment in terms of a significant reduction in serious cardiovascular complications. The results of the two studies are summarised in Table 13.1.

These results, which were supported by uncontrolled studies (Breckenridge, Dollery & Parry, 1970), were interpreted as showing benefit conferred by treating severe hypertension, and it soon became accepted that people with sustained diastolic (phase V) pressures of over 110 mm Hg should be treated. It was assumed that women would benefit in the same way as men but in Hamilton's trial the benefit had been restricted to men; in women there had been no convincing evidence of any overall reduction in cardiovascular events. In the Veterans trial no women had been included.

In the VA trial patients were initially admitted into hospital and only those men whose diastolic (V) pressures averaged 90–129 mm Hg during the 4th to 6th day in hospital were considered for the study. Following the time in hospital there was a 2 to 4 month run-in period when each received placebo tablets to check their compliance. Almost half were excluded at this stage either because they were insufficiently compliant in their tablet taking, or because their diastolic pressures settled outside the trial range. So the VA trial included only well motivated men in whom high pressures were sustained over a prolonged pre-trial period.

The second report from the VA study was published in 1970 and was the first which claimed to deal with the problems of mild

Table 13.1. *The results of two randomised controlled trials for the treatment of severe hypertension*

| Criteria for admission | Hamilton, Thompson & Wisniewski (1964) DBP (IV) >110 mm Hg No complications | | | | Veterans Administration Study Group (1967) (Part 1) DBP (V) 115–129 mm Hg With or without complications | |
| | Men | | Women | | Men | |
	Treated	Controls	Treated	Controls	Treated	Controls
N of patients	22		39		143	
N	10	12	20	19	73	70
Strokes	—	4	3	3	1	3
MI or sudden death	—	1	1	2	—	3
Cardiac failure	—	2	—	3	—	2
Renal failure	—	—	1	—	1	3
Other	—	1	1	—	1	3[a]
Total complications	—	8	5	8	2	14[a]

[a] Excluding 9 who developed 'terminating' fundal changes and 3 with 'terminating' BP changes.

Table 13.2. *The results of the second Veterans Administration*
trial (1970)

Criteria for admission	DBP(V) 90–114 mm Hg Men	
N of patients	380	
	Treated	Controls
N	186	194
Strokes	5	20
MI or sudden death	11	13
Cardiac failure	—	11
Renal failure	—	3
Other	6	9
Total complications	22	56

hypertension (Veterans Administration Co-operative Study Group, 1970). It was a carefully conducted study which set the stage for, and influenced the design of, several later trials but its relevance to mild hypertension, as encountered by family practitioners, has not been accepted outside the USA.

The main results of this second part of the VA trial are summarised in Table 13.2. The rate of occurrence of serious cardiovascular events was high. Among 194 untreated control men, who were followed for an average period of 3.3 years, 56 trial-terminating events occurred; they included 20 strokes, 13 episodes of coronary heart disease, 11 cases of cardiac failure and 4 of 'accelerated' hypertension. Some years later Wilhelmsen, Berglund and Wedel (1979) concluded that the cardiovascular mortality reported in this second part of the VA trial corresponded with that associated with blood pressures of 205–225/ 120–124 mm Hg, as measured in their own epidemiological studies in Sweden. Only 1.5% of middle-aged men in Sweden have pressures at that level; they are not considered to have 'mild hypertension'.

By the time the MRC trial was completed in 1985 the results of several other major trials had been reported. Five of them were very relevant in as much as they included patients with mild hypertension. These were the US Public Health Service Study (USPHS), the Australian National Blood Pressure Study (ANBPS), the US Hypertension Detection and Follow-Up Program (HDFP), the Oslo trial and the International Prospective Primary Prevention Study in Hypertension (IPPPSH).

Some features of the designs of the six more relevant trials, the five mentioned above and the MRC trial, limit their comparability. All were randomised controlled trials but only four of them compared treated with untreated control groups (USPHS, ANBPS, MRC and the Oslo Study).

Those who planned HDFP were influenced by the VA trial results to consider it unethical to include an untreated control group; it was therefore a comparison of groups receiving two different systems of medical (including antihypertensive) care. In one group free care was provided in clinics which were mostly linked with University departments. This was the 'Stepped Care' group, named after the manner in which drug regimes were introduced in steps in an organised way. In the other group people were referred back to their normal sources of medical care – the 'Referred Care' group.

IPPPSH, likewise, did not include an untreated group. It was a large randomised double-blind trial in which over 6000 men and women with uncomplicated hypertension (DBP V 100 – 125 mm Hg) were entered into a study lasting 3–5 years; over 25 000 person-years of observation were accumulated. Half the patients were already on antihypertensive treatment at entry to the study so in general IPPPSH dealt with moderately severely affected people. At the start of the IPPPSH trial patients were assigned randomly to groups receiving either slow-release oxprenolol (160 mg tablets) or placebo tablets of identical appearance. These regimens could form the only treatments given or the initial steps in treatment where any antihypertensive drug other than a beta-blocker could be added, as necessary. The aim of the scheme was to evaluate the effect of using oxprenolol in antihypertensive treatment regimes.

Two of these trials, USPHS and the Oslo trial, were unfortunately too small to have had any chance of showing significant benefit in terms of reduced morbidity or mortality. HDFP, though a valuable study of importance to the USA, compared two systems of medical care neither of which had a close counterpart in other countries.

The Australian trial was a placebo-controlled, single-blind study which was planned to be comparable with the MRC trial. It was stopped when the average follow-up was just over four years; the results at that stage showed an overall benefit just significant at the 5% level. It would not have been easy, or desirable, to attempt to pool results from the two studies because of minor differences in procedures between them.

No single trial can provide all the answers. The different trials had varying aims, used different entry and exclusion criteria, and recruited populations which differed in major ways. Some of their features are compared in Table 13.3. The different crude mortality rates in the control groups are shown in Table 13.4. Despite their differences something can be learnt from an examination of where their results were consistent and where they were inconsistent.

Table 13.3. A comparison of the features of four treatment trials for mild hypertension: the US Hypertension Detection and Follow-up Program (Stratum 1), the Australian National Blood Pressure Study, the MRC trial and the International Prospective Primary Prevention Study in Hypertension

	HDFP	ANBPS	MRC	IPPPSH
No. of subjects	7825	3427	17 354	6357
Person-years of observation	38 178	13 859	85 572	21 267
Per cent men	55	63	52	50
Age range (y)	30–69	30–69	35–64	40–64
DBP(V) range (mm Hg)	90–104	95–109	90–109	100–125
Comparison groups	Stepped Care/ Referred Care	Active/placebo	Thiazide β-blocker Placebo	β-blocker Non β-blocker

Table 13.4. Crude mortality rates per 1000 in four hypertension trials

	HDFP[a]		ANBPS		MRC			IPPPSH	
	Stepped Care	Referred Care	Active	Placebo	Thiazide	β-blocker	Placebo	β-blocker	Non-β-blocker
All causes	12.1	15.3	3.6	5.1	6.0	5.5	5.9	8.3	8.8
All cardiovascular	6.4	8.7	1.1	2.6	3.3	3.0	3.3	4.1	5.4
Cerebrovascular	0.9	1.6	0.4	0.9	0.2	0.6	0.6	0.4	0.8
MI	4.5	5.6	0.7	1.6	2.8	2.2	2.3	3.1	3.6
Non-cardiovascular	5.7	6.6	2.4	2.5	2.8	2.5	2.7	4.7	4.4

[a] Stratum 1.

The evidence concerning stroke prevention

Stroke incidence was reduced in all the placebo controlled studies. The data are not poolable, and the results seem to vary markedly between studies but the consistent benefit is convincing (Table 13.5). The average benefit conferred in the previously reported trials, 44%, corresponds closely with the overall benefit observed in the MRC trial, 45%; it is less than the 66% benefit seen in the MRC's thiazide-treated group.

In the IPPPSH trial the stroke rates in the beta-blocker and the non-beta-blocker groups were almost identical. In the former, 45 strokes occurred, and in the latter, 46, giving rates of 3.5 and 3.6 per 1000 person-years respectively. These rates are about 40% higher than those of untreated controls in the MRC trial and about 150% higher than the treated patients in the MRC trial, and presumably result from the differences in the criteria for acceptance into the two studies.

Within trials there is some evidence that the greater the risk of stroke the greater the potential absolute benefit from treatment. In the Australian trial, which entered people with diastolic pressures of 95–109 mm Hg, the stroke benefit was greater in those with entry pressures over 100 mm Hg. HDFP showed (in its 3 strata according to entry diastolic pressure) that – after standardising for age – the higher the diastolic pressure the greater the risk of stroke and the greater the absolute benefit of treatment (Fig. 13.1). HDFP also showed increasing stroke risks and increasing benefits of treatment with increase in age, after standardisation for blood pressure (Fig. 13.2). The MRC trial also showed greater risks and greater absolute

Table 13.5. *The stroke benefit in randomised controlled trials*

Trial		Fatal and non-fatal strokes		
		Treated	Controls	% reduction
Hamilton et al.	1964	3	7	57
VA trial				
(1) DBP 115–129 mm Hg	1967	1	4	75
(2) DBP 90–114 mm Hg	1970	1	13	92
US Public Health Service	1977	1	6	83
HDFP[a]	1979	102	158	35
Australian trial	1980	13	22	41
Helgeland Oslo trial	1980	—	5	100
Total		121	215	44

[a] HDFP: Treated = Stepped Care group, Controls = Referred Care group.

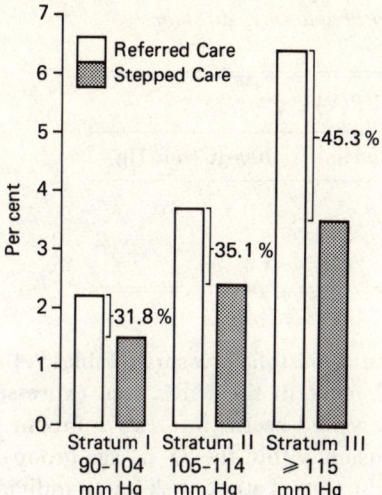

Fig. 13.1. *The 5-year incidence per 1000 person-years of fatal and non-fatal strokes according to entry diastolic pressure, for Stepped Care and Referred Care participants in the US Hypertension Detection and Follow-up Program, adjusted for age, sex and race. (Source: JAMA.* 1982, **247**, 633.)

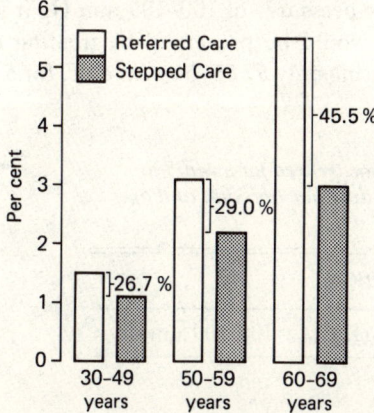

Fig. 13.2. *The 5-year incidence per 1000 person-years of fatal and non-fatal strokes according to age, for Stepped Care participants in the US Hypertension Detection and Follow-up Program, adjusted for race, sex and diastolic pressure. (Source: JAMA.* 1982, **247**, 633.)

Table 13.6. *Incidence of stroke per 1000 patient-years in untreated control subjects in the MRC trial, according to entry diastolic pressure and age. Both sexes together*

	Entry DBP(V)	
Age at entry (y)	<100 mm Hg	100–109 mm Hg
35–44	0.4	1.0
45–54	1.4	2.7
55–64	3.0	5.6

benefits the greater the entry diastolic pressure (Tables 9.4 and 9.5).

Although the stroke benefit in the MRC trial expressed as the proportion of events prevented seems impressive (about 45%, for those with mild hypertension within the 35–64 age-group), it could also be expressed as a reduction of stroke risk for an individual from 0.0025 to 0.0014 per annum, or as one stroke prevented in 5 years as a result of treating 175 mild hypertensives of the type recruited to the trial.

Within the 90–109 mm Hg DEP(V) range of the MRC trial there was no significant difference in the *proportion* of strokes prevented by treatment between those with pressures at the top and at the lower part of the range. But there was a considerable difference in the incidence of strokes not only according to entry pressure but also according to age (Table 13.6) and therefore amongst the older subjects with the higher pressures an opportunity for conferring a larger *absolute* stroke benefit in those at higher risk, as shown from the trial data in Table 13.7. For those with entry pressures of 100–109 mm Hg it would be expected that one stroke would be prevented by treating only 118 45–54-year-olds or by treating only 57 55–64-year olds, for 5 years.

Table 13.7. *The number of patients to be treated for 5 years to prevent one stroke, according to entry diastolic pressure and age (MRC trial data)*

	Entry DBP	
Age (y)	<100 mm Hg	100–109 mm Hg
35–44		500
45–54	400	118
55–64	286	57
35–64	500	95

Table 13.8. *The incidence of stroke per 1000 person-years of observation in men and women, according to systolic pressure as recorded at the 6-month follow-up visit, and randomised treatment group (MRC trial data)*

6-month Systolic pressure (mm Hg)	Bendrofluazide group				Propranolol group				Placebo group			
	Men		Women		Men		Women		Men		Women	
	N	Rate	N	Rate	N	Rate	N	Rate	N	Rate	N	Rate
<135	2	0.4	2	0.4	5	1.0	5	1.3	4	0.7	7	1.2
135–144	1	0.5	1	0.4	3	1.3	2	1.1	9	2.0	8	1.9
145–154	2	1.3	1	1.5	5	2.3	3	2.1	11	2.3	8	1.9
155 and over	4	3.1	3	3.3	12	6.4	4	1.4	33	5.2	20	3.3

If stroke risk were determined solely by age, and by current systolic pressure level we would expect that its incidence would be the same in patients of the same age with the same levels of systolic pressure whether they were on antihypertensive treatment or not. It would be surprising if a blood pressure held down by pharmacological means were associated with the same risk as that in a person whose pressure was at the same level without treatment, and the Australian trial found that for all cardiovascular end-points the complication rate did not quite fall to that of untreated subjects at similar levels.

Table 13.8 shows the stroke incidence in the MRC trial, according to randomised treatment and systolic pressure as recorded at the 6-month follow-up visit. Among men and women treated with pro-pranolol the treated blood pressure level seems to reflect the stroke risk of controls with the same pressures, and the stroke benefit conferred by propranolol is therefore likely to be due solely to the increase in the numbers of people with systolic pressures controlled at lower levels. But for those being treated with the thiazide, and especially those whose 6-month systolic pressures were below 155 mm Hg, the drug appears to confer *greater* benefit than can be attributed to its blood pressure-lowering properties. This surprising finding seems to be one of the important, if unexplained, results of the study.

The evidence concerning CHD prevention

So far as the results for myocardial infarction are concerned, the findings of the relevant trials are summarised in Table 13.9.

There were only 3 coronary thromboses among the treated and 3 among the controls in Hamilton's trial. The first VA trial recorded just 1 sudden death, and 2 MIs in the placebo group, but none in actively treated people. Clearly it is not possible to generalise from such small numbers.

In the second VA study, in which 12 non-fatal MIs were reported, 7 occurred in treated and 5 in control subjects. There were also 12 sudden deaths, 4 among the treated, 8 in controls. No benefit in coronary events was suggested. In USPHS there were 7 MIs and 1 sudden death among the treated, 6 MIs and 1 sudden death in controls. In the Oslo study too, the effect of treatment on MI rates did not appear beneficial; there were 8 non-fatal MIs in treated people and the same number in control subjects, and there were 6 sudden or MI deaths in the treated compared with 2 in the control group.

ANBPS also showed no overall evidence of a treatment-associated reduction in MIs with 33 events in both the treated and control groups. The distribution of fatal events, however, differed from that

Table 13.9. *The effects of treatment for mild hypertension on coronary events in various trials*

Trial	Sudden deaths or fatal MIs		Non fatal CHD events		Total	
	Treated	Controls	Treated	Controls	Treated	Controls
Placebo-controlled trials						
Veterans administration (Part II)	4	8	7	5	11	13
USPHS	1	1	7	6	8	7
Oslo	6	2	8	8	14	10
ANBPS	5	11	28	22	33	33
MRC	106	97	116	137	222	234
Total	122	119	166	178	288	297
Non-placebo-controlled						
HDFP (Stratum 1)	30	56				
MRFIT (hypertensives)	80	79				
Total	110	135				

in the USPHS and Oslo studies, with 5 fatal MIs in treated but 11 in controls.

HDFP, which dealt only with fatal events, reported a 15% benefit in MI rates associated with treatment: 86 deaths due to CHD occurred in 'Stepped Care' participants and 107 in 'Referred Care' subjects.

IPPPSH showed little difference between the two treatment groups either in the rates for sudden death (2.9 and 2.7 per 1000 person-years in the beta-blocker and non-beta-blocker groups respectively) or in the rates for all MIs (4.7 and 5.7 per 1000 person-years respectively). Though these rates were only about half the rates expected by the trial organisers it is not possible to give any reliable estimate of the benefit conferred by treatment in either group. The rates were again considerably higher than those observed in the untreated controls in the MRC trial.

In the MRC trial there was no overall difference in MI rates between treated and control subjects; there was a small treatment-associated increase in fatal events, and a small treatment-associated reduction in non-fatal events (Table 13.9). Nor was there any suggestion of overall benefit associated with either of the two drugs considered separately. It was only when sub-groups of the population were examined that the data suggested differences between treatment groups, with lower rates for sudden deaths in men in the propranolol than in the bendrofluazide groups, and a reduction in all coronary events in male non-smokers (Table 13.10).

IPPPSH and the MRC trial are the only hypertension trials to date which have reported on their experience with beta-blockers and their findings are in accord in several important ways. The results of the two studies can be directly compared only to the extent that each included 2 actively treated groups, one with and one without a beta-blocker.

In both trials the cerebrovascular and cardiac event rates were doubled or more than doubled in smokers, and the incidence of cardiac end points was lower in non-smokers than in smokers in the groups treated with a beta-blocker. In both studies the outcome of treatment appeared to be influenced by smoking status (Figs. 13.3 and 13.4), and each trial independently detected significant interaction between smoking and the type of drug used which affected the incidence of cardiovascular events.

Clearly further confirmation of the value of beta-blocker therapy in the prevention of CHD in non-smokers will be needed. Before the results of these two studies were available, only the HDFP findings offered any hope that antihypertensive treatment might have some impact in preventing CHD and, for the reasons given above, it was not possible to extrapolate from the HDFP experience. There is, how-

Table 13.10. *The incidence of coronary events (per 1000 person-years) in sub-groups of the MRC trial in men and women*

	Men						Women					
	Smokers		Non-smokers		Total		Smokers		Non-smokers		Total	
	N	Rate	N	Rate	N	Rate	N	Rate	N	Rate	N	Rate
Bendrofluazide												
Fatal: sudden	14	4.1	15	2.0	29	2.7	1	0.4	3	0.4	4	0.4
non-sudden	8	2.4	13	1.7	21	1.9	3	1.1	2	0.3	5	0.5
Non-fatal	21	6.2	28	3.7	49	4.5	10	3.6	1	0.1	11	1.1
Total	43	12.7	56	7.4	99	9.1	14	5.1	6	0.8	20	2.0
Propranolol												
Fatal: sudden	5	1.6	7	0.9	12	1.1[++]	3	1.1	1	0.1	4	0.4
non-sudden	12	3.7	14	1.8	26	2.4	3	1.1	2	0.3	5	0.5
Non-fatal	28	8.4	18	2.3	46	4.1	6	2.2	3	0.4	9	0.9
Total	45	13.8	39	5.0[*]	84	7.6	12	4.5	6	0.8	18	1.7
Placebo												
Fatal: sudden	18	2.8	23	1.5	41	1.9	3	0.6	1	0.1	4	0.2
non-sudden	16	2.5	30	1.9	46	2.1	4	0.7	2	0.1	6	0.3
Non-fatal	49	7.3	63	4.1	112	5.1	12	2.2	12	0.8	24	1.0
Total	83	12.6	116	7.5	199	9.0	19	3.5	15	1.0	34	1.5

[++] Rate significantly lower than that in bendrofluazide group ($P = 0.01$).
[*] Rate significantly lower than that in placebo group ($P = 0.05$).

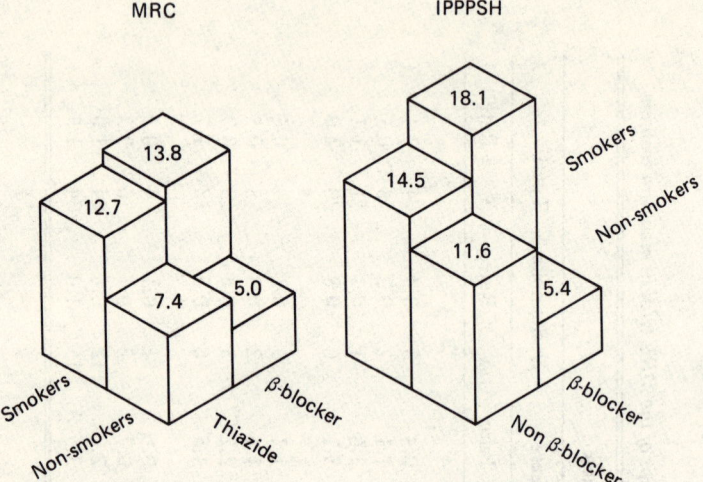

Fig. 13.3. *The incidence per 1000 person-years of coronary events in men in the MRC and IPPPSH trials, according to smoking status and type of active anti-hypertensive treatment.*

ever, encouraging evidence that beta-blockers may be effective in the secondary prevention of myocardial infarction in those who have survived a first attack (May, Eberlin, Furberg *et al.*, 1982). This latter result had always seemed surprising in view of the lack of any overall suggestion in the MRC trial results of a primary preventive effect of beta-blocker treatment. Only when the MRC results were analysed in terms of smoking status did the apparently conflicting findings on primary and secondary prevention make sense. The survivors of MIs are in general non-smokers after their illnesses.

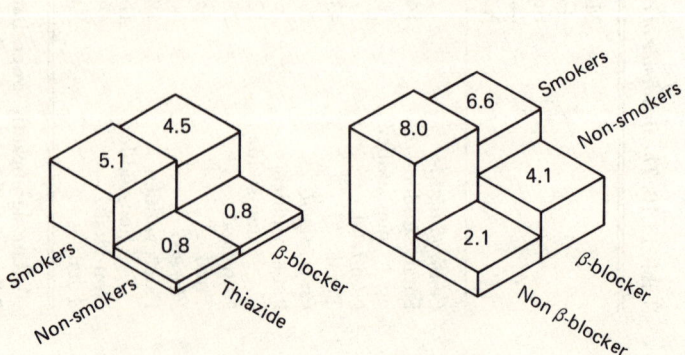

Fig. 13.4. *As for Fig. 13.3, but for women.*

The evidence concerning total mortality

Only the larger trials, of course, provide any indication of the impact of antihypertensive therapy on total mortality. Hamilton's study, the Veterans Administration investigations, USPHS, and the Oslo trial were all too small to do so. In the Australian trial, 25 deaths occurred in the actively treated group and 35 in the controls; MIs, strokes, and other cardiovascular deaths were all reduced in association with active treatment. Seventeen deaths were attributed to causes unconnected with cardiovascular disease in each of the treatment and control groups (Table 13.11).

In HDFP the overall reduction in mortality associated with stepped care was 17%; cardiovascular mortality was reduced by 19%, non-cardiovascular mortality by 14%. In Stratum 1 (DBP at entry 90–104 mm Hg) the corresponding figures were 26% and 13%. This finding, where the relative benefit was higher in those at least risk, seems at first sight to be biologically implausible; it was explained as probably the result of treatment in the Referred Care group having been carried out more assiduously in the more severe hypertensives than in those with less severe disease.

In HDFP the benefits from the better treatment were not shared equally between the two main ethnic groups. In the Stepped Care

Table 13.11. *The incidence of trial end-points per 1000 person-years of observation in the Australian National Blood Pressure Study*

End-point event	Active 6991 person-years		Placebo 6868 person-years	
	N	Rate	N	Rate
Fatal				
MI	5		11	
Stroke	3		6	
All cardiovascular	8	1.1	18	2.6*
Non-cardiovascular	17	2.4	17	2.4
Non-fatal				
MI	28		22	
Other CHD	65		76	
Stroke	10		16	
Other[a]	10		19	
All cardiovascular	113	16.2	133	19.4
All end-points	138	19.7	168	24.5*

* $P < 0.05$.
[a] Other includes transient ischaemic attack, retinopathy, cardiac and renal failure.

group 77% of the mortality reduction occurred in black people who constituted only 44% of the study population. Although the difference in mortality between the Stepped Care and the Referred Care groups has been shown to be significantly and independently related to the differences in treated blood pressure levels during the course of the study (Hardy and Hawkins, 1982), it has not been possible to distinguish the size of the benefit due to the better general medical care from that specifically due to the antihypertensive care given. It would, however, be surprising if better medical care, on its own, could achieve a 17% reduction in all-causes mortality.

The MRC trial results were similar to those of the Australian trial (Table 13.11). There was no real suggestion of a reduction in non-cardiovascular deaths as a result of antihypertensive treatment with either of the two types of drug. This difference between the HDFP results and those of the Australian and British studies cannot be explained by differences in blood pressure control during the trials; in that respect the trials seem to have been similar.

The value of antihypertensive treatment
for those with target organ damage

The Hypertension Detection and Follow-up Program had found that the presence of target organ damage in the Stratum 1 (90–104 mm Hg) group of their study was associated with a three- to five-fold increase in mortality. End-organ damage seemed not only to increase the risk but also to diminish the power of treatment to reduce mortality (Table 13.12). [Note: End-organ damage included history of MI, stroke, intermittent claudication, angina pectoris or an elevated serum creatinine (>1.70 mg/dl).] HDFP also showed for its 90–104 mm Hg group without major target organ damage a 19% higher CHD death rate for the Stepped Care than the Referred Care group if there had been ECG abnormalities present at entry.

Another large American study, the Multiple Risk Factor Intervention Trial (MRFIT) also reported results relevant to the question of target organ damage. MRFIT (Multiple Risk Factor Intervention Trial Research Group, 1982) was designed to determine the value of intervention on the multiple factors which put people at high risk for coronary heart disease and recruited men with enhanced risk – smokers, hypercholesterolaemic and hypertensive subjects. Their risks were usually compounded by the presence of two or more of these risk factors. Participants in MRFIT were allocated at random to groups receiving 'Special Intervention' against coronary risk factors (SI) or 'Usual Care' (UC) and followed for a period of 7 years.

Table 13.12. 5-year all-causes mortality rate in 'Stepped Care' and 'Referred Care' groups, according to presence or absence of end-organ damage.[a] US Hypertension Detection and Follow-up Program, Stratum 1 excluding those on treatment at entry to the trial

End-organ damage	Stepped Care			Referred Care			Reduction in mortality %
	Sample size	N	Rate per 100	Sample size	N	Rate per 100	
Absent	2619	106	4.0	2703	151	5.6	28.6
Present	287	48	16.7	251	44	17.5	4.6

[a] End-organ damage = previous MI, stroke, intermittent claudication, ECG LVH, or serum creatinine greater than 1.7 mg/dl.

Table 13.13. *Coronary deaths, and coronary mortality rates per 100 person-years of observation, according to hypertensive status and ECG abnormality at entry to the trial. US Multiple Risk Factor Intervention Trial*

	Special intervention		Usual care	
	N	Rate	N	Rate
Normotensive				
ECG normal	24	13.2	30	16.1
ECG abnormal	11	18.6	15	25.7
Total	35	14.5	45	18.4
Hypertensive				
ECG normal	44	15.8	58	20.7
ECG abnormal	36	29.2	21	17.7
Total	80	19.9	79	19.8

Among its nearly 13 000 participants were 8000 men with hypertension (DBP(V) 90 mm Hg or more) at entry. The Special Intervention for those who were hypertensive included a programme of 'stepped' drug treatment starting with hydrochlorothiazide or chlorthalidone. In the trial neither total mortality nor CHD mortality was significantly reduced in the SI group compared with the UC group. One possible explanation for this lack of benefit was that some aspect of the intervention programme had a deleterious effect on mortality in some sub-groups and *post hoc* analyses were undertaken to explore this. It was found that SI was more effective in reducing CHD mortality in non-hypertensive than in hypertensive men, and in those without rather than in those with ECG abnormalities in the baseline ECGs (Table 13.13). Although the most obvious cause of the difference in mortality between the SI and UC groups with abnormal ECGs was the unexpectedly low rate in the Usual Care group, a finger was pointed towards diuretic treatment as a possible cause of the higher rate in the SI group.

These findings prompted further studies by both the HDFP and the MRFIT investigators. In a group of HDFP subjects who were selected to be comparable with those reported from MRFIT, the HDFP investigators found reduced mortality in the more-intensive treatment group (SC) than in the less-intensive treatment group (RC) in those without baseline ECG abnormalities. This was true for all-causes, cardiovascular and CHD mortality. Among those with ECG abnormalities all-causes mortality and cardiovascular mortality were also reduced, but there was no CHD benefit. But for white men the mortality for men with baseline ECG abnormalities was actually

Table 13.14. *Five-year all-causes, all cardiovascular and coronary mortality rates in white men in the Stepped Care and Referred Care groups according to the presence or absence of ECG abnormalities. US Hypertension Detection and Follow-up Program, Stratum 1, excluding those on antihypertensive treatment at entry, and those with major organ-system abnormalities*

	Stepped Care		Referred Care	
Without ECG abnormalities	777		745	
All causes	22	28.3	29	38.9
All cardiovascular	11	14.2	12	16.1
Coronary	8	10.3	11	14.8
With ECG abnormalities	313		318	
All causes	21	67.1	23	72.3
All cardiovascular	14	44.7	12	37.7
Coronary	11	35.1	7	22.0

adverse for all cardiovascular and for CHD deaths (Table 13.14). The numbers were, however, small and the differences not statistically significant; the HDFP workers concluded that their findings offered no support for the hypothesis raised in MRFIT that intensive diuretic therapy may increase the mortality rate of hypertensive patients with resting ECG abnormalities (Hypertension Detection and Follow-up Program Co-operative Research Group 1984).

Subsequent analyses of the MRFIT data were undertaken (Multiple Risk Factor Intervention Trial Research Group, 1985). The MRFIT investigators acknowledged that a possible explanation of the difference in outcome was an unexpectedly low CHD mortality among UC participants with ECG abnormalities. But within-group analysis revealed interaction between ECG abnormalities and diuretic treatment in the SI group, with the risk of CHD death for men prescribed diuretics relative to men not prescribed diuretics estimated at 3.34 in those with ECG abnormalities, and at 0.95 in men without such abnormalities. Most of the excess deaths were sudden (Table 13.15) and the majority were associated with hydrochlorothiazide rather than with chlorothalidone.

These findings were viewed with some scepticism. They were based on a heterogeneous group of ECG abnormalities, and applied to resting ECGs but not to exercise ECGs (Multiple Risk Factor Intervention Trial Research Group, 1985). A formal request from the US National Heart Lung and Blood Institute was received by the MRC co-ordinating centre asking for analyses similar to those undertaken by MRFIT, using data from the MRC trial. The analyses described in Chapters 7 and 11 were already nearing completion. Did they confirm or did they refute the MRFIT and HDFP findings?

Table 13.15. *Coronary deaths, and coronary mortality rates per 1000 person-years of observation, according to the presence or absence of ECG abnormalities at rest, at baseline. US Multiple Risk Factor Intervention Trial*

	Special intervention		Usual care	
Without ECG abnormalities	2785		2808	
Myocardial infarction	15	5.4	14	5.0
Sudden death within 1 h	19	6.8	23	8.2
Sudden death 1–24 h	9	3.2	16	5.7
Other	1	0.3	5	1.8
Total	44	15.8	58	20.7
With ECG abnormalities	1233		1185	
Myocardial infarction	9	7.3	8	6.8
Sudden death within 1 h	21	17.0	8	6.8
Sudden death 1–24 h	4	3.2	5	4.2
Other	2	1.6	0	0.0
Total	36	29.2	21	17.7

The MRC trial showed an increased incidence of ECG changes compatible with infarction in those treated with the thiazide and evidence that such ECG changes were significantly associated with increased CHD morbidity and mortality compared with those without such changes. In this respect they were similar to the same ECG changes seen in those on the β blocker and on the placebo. Treatment with the thiazide, however, was not associated with any significant increase in CHD events as a whole.

Careful assessment of the results of the HDFP, MRFIT and MRC trials provides no strong evidence that thiazide treatment of mild hypertension increases the risk of cardiac complications in those with ECG evidence of heart involvement.

ECG abnormalities in IPPPSH were classified as either pressure-related or ischaemia-related. Neither of these two groups seemed to have special predictive value for the outcome of treatment in either the beta-blocker or the non-beta-blocker groups though their value as indicators of end-organ involvement including the development of hypertensive heart disease, was confirmed.

The results of the IPPPSH and the MRC trials were obtained independently and published almost at the same time. Their similarity in demonstrating interaction between cigarette smoking and treatment benefits adds conviction that the finding is a real one. In some respects each trial can be considered to have provided the hypothesis which the other was able to test and confirm, but further confirmation is still needed.

If the β-blocker benefit in non-smokers were to be confirmed, and if, as seems likely, the CHD risk of ex-smokers quickly reverts to that of non-smokers, the impact of mild hypertension could be markedly diminished for those who are at risk and willing to accept the necessary changes in life-style.

14 Commentary

At the time when the first results of the trial were being published the Working Party thought that it would be wiser to avoid giving its own interpretation of their therapeutic implications.

Some of us thought that those who were most closely involved in the planning and conduct of the study, and in the collection and analysis of the data it produced, were unlikely to be able to provide a dispassionate and objective opinion on its results, and that it was the Working Party's job just to collect the evidence and report it. The medical world would then decide how that evidence, together with evidence from other sources, should influence practice.

This view was not shared by everyone. Others thought that though the Working Party might have inflated opinions on the value of the trial they nevertheless had had longer to consider the implications of its results than anyone else, and for that reason should have advice worth offering. There was also a feeling that less-specialised doctors could reasonably expect advice from hypertension 'experts'. Whether the decision not to make recommendations was correct or not, it probably contributed to the rather negative coverage by the lay press following a press conference arranged to coincide with the publication (Prentice, 1985; Veitch, 1985).

In this final chapter we give some of our own interpretations of the results and review those features of the trial which we think have taught us, and therefore might teach others, a useful lesson. This includes some discussion of the unforeseen ethical problems which cropped up during the 12-year course of the trial and how, in the light of our own experience, we would suggest changes in the rôles of committees appointed to advise on such issues.

The overall balance-sheet of the trial results

The starkest and simplest account of the trial results would be to state merely that they showed only that treatment with bendrofluazide and propranolol, in the doses used, reduced the incidence of strokes without reducing all-causes mortality, and was without significant overall effect on coronary heart disease. In achieving this the treatment also prevented the progression from mild to more severe grades of hypertension in about one-eighth of the people treated.

Part of the problem in interpreting the trial stems from the fact that the benefit among the treated is unevenly distributed. It varies with age, with sex and with the type of antihypertensive drug; it also differs between smokers and non-smokers.

Nevertheless some generalisations can be made. For any given level of blood pressure the risk of stroke is much less in younger than in older people; if we disregard other considerations there is a stronger case for treating older than younger patients, within the age range considered in the trial. The cardiovascular risks in general are greater in men than in women; this is true of stroke as well as coronary heart disease; at any given age there is, if we disregard other considerations, a stronger case for treating men than women. And the risks and the benefits of treatment are greater the higher the pressure; at any age and in either sex the higher the pressure the stronger the case for drug treatment.

But we could use other information from the trial to dictate policy. Neither bendrofluazide nor propranolol showed any indication that they conferred protection against coronary heart disease in smokers. On the other hand bendrofluazide was remarkably effective in preventing stroke in smokers. One element of a treatment policy might therefore be to treat all mildly hypertensive smokers with a thiazide.

Propranolol seemed to be as effective as bendrofluazide in preventing stroke in non-smoking men; in addition it prevented a number of coronary events. Another element of a treatment policy might be to treat all non-smoking men with a β-blocker.

Although treatment reduced the number of strokes in non-smoking women there was a worrying suggestion in the trial that overall mortality was increased by treatment in this group. Non-smoking mildly hypertensive women are at low risk of cardiovascular complications and a third element of a treatment policy might therefore be to withhold drug treatment in this group.

Applying these three policies together (even ignoring questions of age and blood pressure level within the range) would be expected to cause a reduction of 52% for strokes, 12% for coronary events and 21% for all deaths in a population of the same age and sex structure, and with the same smoking habits, as in the trial population. Recommendations based on such analysis could form simple and easily administered guidelines which might serve until better data (or better drugs) are available.

But to recommend such a policy would mean advocating drug treatment for all adults aged 35–64 with diastolic pressures of 90–109 mm Hg, with the exception of non-smoking women, and on the present evidence we do not think that is warranted. In our view a major public health approach towards the treatment of all 35–64-year-old people with diastolic pressures sustained in the 90–109 mm Hg range could not be justified because so many would be treated for the benefit of so few, and therefore the costs both in monetary terms and in terms of side-effects would be too great.

Some people may feel that stroke is such a serious complication of hypertension and so preventable, particularly with thiazides (which in the trial data reduced the overall incidence by 67%), that for this alone treatment would be warranted. But even for stroke, where the benefits are clear-cut, they need to be balanced against the costs in terms of adverse reactions, and the case for such a policy would be stronger if treatment were restricted to (say) those over 50 years old with diastolic pressures of 100 mm Hg or more. Younger and less-hypertensive subjects seem at too low a risk of stroke for drug treatment to be a practicable approach for them.

Although a mass approach to the problem of treating mild hypertension seems inappropriate, groups of patients can be identified who are at sufficiently increased risk to warrant treatment. All the present evidence points to the following important risk factors:

    (a) the level of pre-treated or of treated blood pressure
    (b) cigarette-smoking habits
    (c) increased age
    (d) obesity in men
    (e) raised cholesterol level
    (f) ECG abnormalities suggesting myocardial ischaemia or hypertrophy
    (g) heavy alcohol consumption
    (h) adverse family history.

Advice about the risks of cigarette smoking for those with mild hypertension seems of paramount importance; control of obesity, of serum cholesterol level and of alcohol consumption are also needed whether or not drug treatment is initiated.

Revised guidelines for the treatment of mild hypertension, endorsed at the 4th Mild Hypertension Conference sponsored by WHO and the International Society of Hypertension, recommended that drug treatment be considered for those retaining diastolic pressures of 100 mm Hg after 4 weeks of observation, and that those with pressures above 95 mm Hg after a 3-month observation period should start drug treatment. Mild hypertension was defined as DBP(V) 90–104 mm Hg (WHO/ISH, 1986).

The trial analyses suggested that mild hypertensives with diastolic(V) blood pressures remaining above 100 mm Hg over a period of

4 weeks and those who retained a pressure of 95 mm Hg or more after 3 or 6 months of observation, and especially if male and over the age of 45, did benefit most from treatment. In some patients treatment does not need to be continuous and a period off treatment can be tried provided careful monitoring of blood pressure continues.

Because the cardiovascular risk in mildly hypertensive women is so much lower than that of men, it seems justifiable to withhold treatment altogether from them and merely monitor blood pressure, treating only those whose pressures threaten to exceed the mild-hypertension range. But the regular monitoring of blood pressure levels and control of other risk factors should be an essential element of care in such women so that treatment is started before target-organ damage occurs.

Some of the ethical issues involved

During the course of this trial we became increasingly convinced of the difficulty of specifying from the outset all the questions for which a study of this kind is likely to be able to provide answers. Many of the questions arose from the data as they accumulated, but were none the less important for that.

The first ethical issue concerned the dose of the thiazide which we were using. In 1979, when the trial had already been in progress for about 6 years, the routine monitoring showed the incidence of fatal coronary events to be higher in the bendrofluazide group, in both sexes, than in untreated controls. Coronary events were also running at a higher rate in the men on bendrofluazide than in those on the beta-blocker. At about the same time the Monitoring Committee became aware of the fact that ECG evidence of myocardial infarction and ECG evidence of ventricular ectopic arrhythmias were also both increased in men who were on the thiazide.

The trial's Ethical Committee was informed of these trends and advised that the Working Party should reconsider the dose of bendrofluazide used in the trial.

A special meeting of the Working Party was called. Until that time its members (with the exception of those who served also on the trial's Monitoring Committee), and its Chairman, had been kept completely ignorant of the trends in morbidity and mortality in the different drug groups, but not unreasonably they were unwilling to pronounce on a matter of this importance to the trial without being made fully aware of the underlying facts. They were therefore temporarily 'unblinded' for the relevant sections of the results.

After consideration of the data, and with the knowledge that the adverse ECG trends were only at the margins of statistical significance and were not accompanied by significant differences in the rates of CHD events between the thiazide and control groups, the Working Party thought the trial should continue unchanged. This decision was taken because the Working Party was very unwilling to throw suspicion on a group of drugs of such widespread use unless the evidence for so doing was irrefutable. Even 6 years later when the trial was closed the evidence was still not conclusive; the ECG evidence alone was not enough and the differences in the incidences of events between the thiazide group and controls were not significant.

The next major ethical question came in June 1983 when there was a demonstrable reduction in the stroke rate but no clear evidence of overall benefit. On this occasion the Ethical Committee recommended that the trial be continued 'to obtain further evidence on (a) total mortality, including mortality from myocardial infarction, sudden death, and some non-vascular causes and (b) interactions between treatment and smoking habits'.

In setting up the committees to monitor the trial's progress and to advise on its termination, the Working Party had (rightly or wrongly) retained for itself the executive decision as to whether the trial should be continued or stopped in the light of any recommendations it received. Although from the outset the Working Party had set rules which required the Ethical Committee to inform the Secretary of the Medical Research Council and the Chairman of the Working Party when it was convinced that certain statistical criteria had been met, there had been no intention to restrict either the right of the Ethical Committee to decide for itself what detailed results should be reported, nor when they should be reported, nor what action it should recommend the Working Party to take. Until such detailed results or recommendations were received the Working Party considered it should not be party to the data.

So the Ethical Committee's advice that the trial be continued despite having met statistical criteria which the Working Party believed (in fact wrongly) would stop it, meant that the *de facto* rules governing the trial's monitoring and cessation had altered without the Working Party as a whole knowing that this had occurred, and an additional complication was provided by the overlap between the membership of the Working Party and its Monitoring Committee which meant that some members were aware of the facts while others were kept uninformed. The problems were also accentuated by the overlap in function between the Monitoring and Ethical Committees. The Monitoring Committee advised the co-ordinating centre on analyses, and then decided on the report to be sent to the Ethical Committee; naturally they held views themselves on the propriety or otherwise of continuing the trial. In this kind of situation there should probably be as little overlap as possible between the data gatherers and those who adjudicate on them. Other trialists may learn, as we did, from this experience.

In effect the Chairman of the Working Party asked to see the data on which the recommendation had been made so that he, himself, was in as strong and informed a position as possible to make a decision. He accepted the Ethical Committee's advice and agreed to the trial's continuation. Those members of the Working Party who were not immediately aware of the decision that the trial was to continue, despite having reached a point where they would have imagined that it would be stopped, were soon informed of the position by the Chairman, accepted it with good grace, and said that they would prefer to remain ignorant of all details.

The decision to continue the trial for at least another six months, or possibly until its planned completion at 90 000 person-years of observation, raised a number of interesting issues. What if the significance of the difference in stroke incidence were to diminish? Should we accept the original estimate or that based on the larger quantity of data? The purpose of continuing would be to seek new information, but the credibility of any new findings would be diminished because it would be said (quite rightly) that we had broken our stopping rules in order to have a better chance of obtaining those findings. This loss of credibility would be directly related to the number of newly introduced stopping options; it would be least, though still present, with a simple decision to continue to completion.

It seemed in fact unlikely that continuation of the trial could resolve the question whether active treatment resulted in increased mortality, since there would be too few remaining person-years of observation to be able to demonstrate that even if it were true. The decision to continue preserved at least the original intentions which were to determine the effects of treatment (with two separate regimes or pooled) on strokes, CHD events and total mortality in men and women (separately or combined). One real advantage of continuing would be to reduce the confidence interval around a negative result and this seemed the likeliest outcome with respect to the effects on total mortality. Another would be to obtain maximal information about sub-groups and in particular about the relationship between the effects of the drugs in smokers and non-smokers.

Although the decision was to extend the trial only for periods of six months at a time after each of which the new data were submitted to the Ethical Committee, the trial did in fact continue up to the time of its originally planned completion.

So by February 1985 the experiment was over. Its results were by no means a clear-cut endorsement of the policies some were advocating on the basis of the results of the earlier trials. It was an expensive experiment (by British if not by American standards); but if it helps towards a more rational approach to the treatment of mild hypertension, it may spare a great many people from developing the adverse reactions to drugs which would benefit them little. If it also helps towards a more rational use of drugs by indicating which people with mild hypertension are at increased risk, and how they differ in their response to treatment with the two classes of hypertensive drugs which are still in most common use for mild hypertension today, the trial may indeed save a great deal more than it cost.

Bibliography

Ablad, B., Carlsson, E., Johnsson, G. & Regardh, C-G. (1980). In *Pharmacology of Antihypertensive Drugs*, ed. A. Scriabine, pp. 247–62. New York: Raven Press.

Aho, H., Harmsen, P., Hatano, S., Marquardsen, W., Smirnov, V. E. & Strasser, T. (1980). Cerebrovascular disease in the community; results of a WHO collaborative study. *Bulletin of the World Health Organisation,* **58**, 113–30.

Anonymous. (1980). Mild hypertension. *British Medical Journal,* **280**, 1062–3.

Anonymous. (1980). The pressure to treat. *Lancet,* **1**, 1283–4.

Anonymous. (1980). Millions of mild hypertensives. *British Medical Journal,* **281**, 1024–5.

Australian National Blood Pressure Study Management Committee. (1980). The Australian therapeutic trial in mild hypertension. *Lancet,* **1**, 1261–7.

Breckenridge, A., Dollery, C. T. & Parry, E. H. D. (1970). Prognosis of treated hypertension. Changes in life expectancy and causes of death between 1952 and 1967. *Quarterly Journal of Medicine,* **39**, 411–29.

Brennan, P. J., Greenberg, G., Miall, W. E. & Thompson, S. G. (1982). Seasonal variation in arterial blood pressure. *British Medical Journal,* **285**, 919–23.

Broughton, P. M. G., Holder, R. & Ashby, D. (1986). Long-term trends in biochemical data obtained from two population surveys. *Annals of Clinical Biochemistry,* **23**, 474–86.

Bulpitt, C. J. & Dollery, C. T. (1973). Side effects of hypotensive agents evaluated by a self administered questionnaire. *British Medical Journal,* **3**, 485–90.

Cryer, P. E., Haymond, M. W., Santiago, J. V. & Shah, S. D. (1976). Norepinephrine and epinephrine release and adrenergic mediation of smoking associated haemodynamic and metabolic events. *New England Journal of Medicine,* **295**, 573–7.

Doll, W. R. S. (1983). Prospects for prevention. *British Medical Journal,* **286**, 445–53.

Fox, K. M., Deanfield, J., Selwyn, A., Krikler, S. & Wright, C. (1983). Factors influencing the treatment of chronic stable angina pectoris with nifedipine. *Postgraduate Medical Journal,* **59** (Suppl. 2), 25–9.

Goldberg, D. P., Cooper, B., Eastwood, M. R., Kedward, H. B. & Shepherd, M. (1970). A standardised psychiatric interview for use in community surveys. *British Journal of Preventive and Social Medicine,* **24**, 18–23.

Goldberg, D. P. (1972). *The Detection of Psychiatric Illness by Questionnaire.* London: Oxford University Press.

Greenberg, G. & Thompson, S. G. (1984). The effect of smoking on blood pressure in mild hypertensives, and on their response to antihypertensive treatment. *Journal of Hypertension,* **2**, 553.

Hamilton, M., Thompson, E. N. & Wisniewski, T. K. M. (1964). The role of blood pressure control in preventing complications of hypertension. *Lancet,* **1**, 235–8.

Hardy, R. J. & Hawkins, C. M. (1982). The impact of selected indices of antihypertensive treatment on all-cause mortality. *American Journal of Epidemiology,* **117**, 566–74.

Hata, J., Ogihara, T., Maruyama, A. *et al.* (1982). The seasonal variation of blood pressure in patients with essential hypertension. *Clinical and Experimental Hypertension – Theory and Practice,* **A4**, 341–54.

Helgeland, A. (1980). Treatment of mild hypertension. A five year controlled drug trial. The Oslo Study. *American Journal of Medicine,* **69**, 725–32.

Heller, R. F., Rose, G., Tunstall Pedoe, H. D. & Christie, D. G. S. (1978). Blood pressure measurement in the United Kingdom Heart Disease Prevention Project. *Journal of Epidemiology and Community Health,* **32**, 235–8.

Hiatt, W. R., Wolfel, E. E., Stoll, S. *et al.* (1985). Beta-adrenergic blockade evaluated with epinephrine after placebo, atenolol and nadopol. *Clinical Pharmacology and Therapeutics,* **37**, 2–6.

Higgins, I. T. T., Kannel, W. B. & Dawber, T. R. (1965). The electrocardiogram in epidemiological studies. Reproducibility, validity, and international comparison. *British Journal of Preventive and Social Medicine,* **19**, 53–68.

Holland, O. B., Nixon, J. V. & Kuthnert, L. (1981). Diuretic-induced ventricular ectopic activity. *American Journal of Medicine,* **70**, 762–8.

Hollifield, J. W. & Slaton, P. E. (1980). Cardiac arrhythmias associated with diuretic-induced hypokalaemia and hypomagnesaemia. *Royal Society of Medicine International Congress and Symposium Series,* No. 44, 17–26.

Hypertension Detection and Follow-up Program Cooperative Group. (1979). Five year findings of the hypertension detection and follow-up program. (1). Reduction in mortality of persons with high blood pressure, including mild hypertension. (2). Mortality by race, sex and age. *Journal of the American Medical Association,* **242**, 2562–77.

Hypertension Detection and Follow-up Program Cooperative Research Group. (1982). Five year findings of the hypertension detection and follow-up program. (3). Reduction in stroke incidence among persons with high blood pressure. *Journal of the American Medical Association,* **247**, 633–8.

Hypertension Detection and Follow-up Program Cooperative Research

Group. (1984). The effect of antihypertensive drug treatment on mortality in the presence of resting electrocardiographic abnormalities at baseline: the HDFP experience. *Circulation,* **70**, 996–1003.

IPPPSH Collaborative Group. (1985). Cardiovascular risk and risk factors in a randomised trial of treatment based on a Beta-blocker Oxprenolol: The International Prospective Primary Prevention Study in Hypertension (IPPPSH). *Journal of Hypertension,* **3**, 379–92.

Kannel, W. B., Brand, N., Skinner, J. J., Dawber, T. R. & McNamara, P. M. (1967). The relation of adiposity to blood pressure and development of hypertension. *Annals of Internal Medicine,* **67**, 48–59.

Kornitzer, M., De Backer, G., Dramaix, M. *et al.* (1983). Belgian Heart Disease Prevention Project: incidence and mortality results. *Lancet,* **1**, 1066–70.

Mann, A. H. (1977). The psychological effect of a screening programme and clinical trial upon the participants. *Psychological Medicine,* **7**, 431–8.

Mann, Anthony. (1984). Hypertension: psychological aspects and diagnostic impact in a clinical trial. *Psychological Medicine Monograph 5.* Cambridge: Cambridge University Press.

May, G. S., Eberlin, K. A., Furberg, C. D. *et al.* (1982). Secondary prevention after myocardial infarction – a review of long term trials. *Progress in Cardiovascular Diseases,* **25**, 335–59.

McFate Smith, W. (1979). US Public Health Service Hospitals Cooperative Study Group (1977). Treatment of mild hypertension: results of a ten year intervention trial. *Circulation Research,* **40** (suppl), I, 98–105.

Meade, T. W. (1984). Clotting factors and ischaemic heart disease: the epidemiological evidence. In *Anticoagulants and Myocardial Infarction: A Reappraisal,* ed. T. W. Meade, pp. 91–111. Chichester: Wiley.

Meade, T. W., Mellows, S., Brozovic, M. *et al.* (1986). Haemostatic function and ischaemic heart disease: principal results of the Northwick Park Heart Study. *Lancet,* **2**, 533–7.

Medical Research Council Working Party on Mild to Moderate Hypertension (1977). Randomised controlled trial of treatment for mild hypertension: design and pilot trial. *British Medical Journal,* **1**, 1437–40.

Medical Research Council Working Party on Mild to Moderate Hypertension (1981). Adverse reactions to bendrofluazide and propranolol for the treatment of mild hypertension. *Lancet,* **2**, 539–43.

Medical Research Council Working Party on Mild to Moderate Hypertension (1983). Ventricular extrasystoles during thiazide treatment: substudy of the MRC mild hypertension trial. *British Medical Journal,* **287**, 1249–53.

Medical Research Council Working Party on Mild to Moderate Hypertension (1985). MRC trial of treatment of mild hypertension: principal results. *British Medical Journal,* **291**, 97–104.

Medical Research Council Working Party on Mild to Moderate Hypertension (1986*a*). Dose-response to (1) bendrofluazide and (2) hydrochlorothiazide, and the effect of potassium supplementation on the hypotensive action of bendrofluazide: substudies of the Medical

Research Council's trials of treatment of mild hypertension. *British Medical Journal* (in press).

Medical Research Council Working Party on Mild to Moderate Hypertension (1986*b*). The course of blood pressure in mild hypertensives following withdrawal of long-term antihypertensive treatment. *British Medical Journal*, **293**, 988–92.

Miall, W. E., Bell, R. & Lovell, H. G. (1968). Relation between change in blood pressure and weight. *British Journal of Preventive and Social Medicine*, **22**, 73–80.

Multiple Risk Factor Intervention Trial Research Group (1982). Multiple Risk Factor Intervention Trial. Risk factor changes and mortality results. *Journal of the American Medical Association*, **248**, 1465–77.

Multiple Risk Factor Intervention Trial Research Group (1985) Baseline rest electrocardiographic abnormalities, antihypertensive treatment, and mortality in the Multiple Risk Factor Intervention Trial. *American Journal of Cardiology*, **55**, 1–15.

Multiple Risk Factor Intervention Trial Research Group (1985). Exercise electrocardiogram and coronary heart disease mortality in the Multiple Risk Factor Intervention Trial. *American Journal of Cardiology*, **55**, 16–24.

Office of Population Censuses and Surveys (1981). *Cigarette Smoking: 1972–1980*. London: HMSO GHS 81/82.

Peart, W. S. (1980). The pharmaceutical industry: research and responsibility. *Lancet*, **2**, 465–6.

Prentice, T. (1985). Doubts on blood pressure drugs. *Times* 11th July, p. 7.

Reader, R. Personal Communication.

Relman, A. S. (1980). Mild hypertension: no more benign neglect. *New England Journal of Medicine*, **302**, 293–4.

Rose, G. (1961). Seasonal variation in blood pressure in man. *Nature*, **189**, 235.

Rose, G. (1965). Standardisation of observers in blood pressure measurement. *Lancet*, **1**, 673–4.

Rose, G. A. & Blackburn, H. (1966). *Cardiovascular Population Studies: Methods*. Geneva: World Health Organisation.

Rose, G. A., Holland, W. W. & Crowley, E. A. (1964). A sphygmomanometer for epidemiologists. *Lancet*, **1**, 296–300.

Rose, G., Tunstall Pedoe, H. D. & Heller, R. F. (1983). UK Heart Disease Prevention Project: Incidence and mortality results. *Lancet*, **1**, 1062–6.

Struthers, A. D., Reid, J. L., McLean, K. & Rodger, J. C. (1981). Adrenaline, hypokalaemia and cardiac arrhythmias: effects of beta adrenoceptor antagonists. *Clinical Science*, **62**, 1P–57P.

Trap-Jensen, J., Carlsen, J. E., Lysbo-Svendsen, T. & Christensen, N. J. (1979). Cardiovascular and adrenergic effects of cigarette smoking during immediate non-selective and selective beta adrenoceptor blockage in humans. *European Journal of Clinical Investigation*, **9**, 181–3.

US Department of Health and Human Services. The Health Consequences of Smoking: Cardiovascular Disease. A Report to the Surgeon General.

US Department of Health and Human Services, Public Service Office on Smoking and Health. DHSS Publication No (PHS) 84-50204, 1983, pp. 291–326.

Veitch, A. (1985). Blood pressure treatment ruled out. *Guardian*, 11th July, p. 3.

Veterans Administration Cooperative Study Group. (1967). Effects of treatment on morbidity in hypertension. Results in patients with diastolic blood pressure averaging 115 through 129 mm Hg. *Journal of the American Medical Association,* **202**, 1028–34.

Veterans Administration Cooperative Study Group. (1970). Effects of treatment on morbidity in hypertension. Results in patients with diastolic blood pressures averaging 90 through 114 mm Hg. *Journal of the American Medical Association,* **213**, 1143–52.

Wilhelmsen, L., Berglund, G. & Wedel, H. (1979). Benefits of blood pressure treatment in a general middle-aged male population. In *Mild Hypertension: Natural History and Management*, ed. F. Gross & T. Strasser, pp. 47–56. London: Pitman.

Wilhelmsen, L., Berglund, G., Elmfeldt, D. & Wedel, H. (1981). Beta-blockers versus saluretics in hypertension. *Preventive Medicine,* **10**, 38–49.

World Health Organisation Regional Ofice for Europe. (1976). *Myocardial Infarction Community Registers*. Copenhagen: WHO. (Public Health in Europe No. 5.)

World Health Organisation/International Society of Hypertension Mild Hypertension Liaison Committee. (1982). Trials of the treatment of Mild Hypertension: an interim report. *Lancet,* **1**, 149–56.

World Health Organisation European Collaborative Group. (1983). Multifactorial trial in the prevention of coronary heart disease. (3). Incidence and mortality results. *European Heart Journal,* **4**, 141–7.

World Health Organisation/International Society of Hypertension. (1986). Guidelines for the treatment of Mild Hypertension: memorandum from a WHO/ISH meeting. *Journal of Hypertension*, **4**, 383–6.

Wright, B. M. & Dore, C. F. (1970). A random-zero sphygmomanometer. *Lancet,* **1**, 337–8.

Appendix A
The costs of the trial

Large-scale national therapeutic trials are expensive. As discussed below, extrapolation from the pilot trial experience indicated that the total cost of obtaining the 90 000 person-years of observation required for the definitive trial would amount to £2 000 000 to £2 500 000 spread over a period of about eight years. In assessing whether the information obtained from such a study was likely to be worth this kind of money, it was necessary to consider the expenditure in the context of the national costs of treatment, on the one hand, and the national costs of hospital admissions for strokes and coronary heart attacks on the other.

At the time that the MRC Systems Board was considering the funding for the main phase of the trial it was calculated that the *annual* costs of drugs, alone, were treatment to be given for all 35–64-year-old adults in Britain with sustained diastolic pressures of 90–109 mm Hg, would amount to about £3M with the thiazide or about £17.5M with the beta-blocker.

If the trial were to show treatment to be ineffective, or unwarranted, in this blood-pressure range, the costs of the trial would need to be balanced against the savings which could result from that finding. Already, before the trial was expanded, there was a trend (encouraged by the £2M to £3M spent at that time by the pharmaceutical industry, each year, on advertising antihypertensive drugs in this country), to treat milder degrees of hypertension despite the lack of evidence of the effectiveness of such treatment.

In 1975 about £22M was spent on antihypertensive drugs (excluding diuretics) in the UK. In the US, largely as a result of acceptance of the Veterans Administration Trial results, sales of antihypertensive drugs had risen from US$118M in 1965 to US$383M in 1975). If the MRC trial were to find even a small fraction of the mildly hypertensive population to be best left untreated (and this finding were acted upon), the annual saving in drugs could amount to the total costs of the trial.

At the time the MRC Working Party was seeking the funds for the expansion of the trial, there were about 100 000 hospital admissions for cerebrovascular disease annually, and over 130 000 admissions for ischaemic heart disease. The direct costs to the National Health Service (at 1969 prices) had been estimated by the Office of Health Economics to be £41.9M per annum for cerebrovascular disease and £27.5M per annum for ischaemic heart disease. These costs did not cover out-patient costs or the costs of time lost from work.

If the incidence of either of these major complications of hypertension could be reduced by controlling hypertension more effectively, there could be a major financial saving to set against the increased costs of prevention. The total cost of obtaining the information, by completing the trial, seemed likely to be commensurate with the *annual* potential savings whether the trial produced a positive or a negative result provided there was some responsiveness of the medical profession, and the public, to those results.

The estimate of £2 115 000 for the trial, derived from an extrapolation from pilot trial expenditure (described in Chapter 2) excluded the costs of the accommodation at the coordinating centre, which was part of a Medical Research Council Unit and separately financed; no provision was made for the purchase of trial drugs, which were donated by the manufacturers; and no expenditure on biochemical investigations was required as these were also separately financed.

The estimate for the costs of the main trial, excluding the £81 000 already incurred on the pilot phase, was of the order of £2 035 000. At that time it was thought that the trial would take another eight years to complete. In fact the expenditure was spread over ten years, at a time when inflation was running high. The actual expenditure amounted to £3 204 525, of which £2 325 255 was spent on salaries, and £879 270 on equipment and all other costs.

This figure of £3 204 525 was for the actual expenditure incurred during the financial years 1976/77 to 1985/86. When corrected for inflation to accord with the purchasing power of the pound in 1976/77 (when the estimates were made) it became £2 069 652. The cost of the trial, in terms of the purchasing power of the pound in 1986/87, would be £4 466 500.

Appendix B
MRC treatment trial for mild hypertension

<u>O P E R A T I N G   M A N U A L</u>

Coordinating Centre,
MRC/DHSS Epidemiology and
Medical Care Unit,
Northwick Park Hospital,
Watford Road,
HARROW,
Middx, HA1 3UJ.

Blood Pressure Recording

No strenuous exertion by subject within 10 minutes before measurement.
For 3 minutes (at least) subject should be seated where the measurement
will be made.   All measurements with subject seated; either arm can
be used.   Use random zero instrument (or London School of Hygiene
sphygmomanometer).   If gross discrepancies occur between the two
corrected readings (as occasionally happens if the zero-error is read
when the cuff is improperly deflated etc.), please repeat.

(1) Record systolic, diastolic V (disappearance) to the nearest 2 mm Hg.

(2) Record zero error (to nearest 1 mm) after making sure the valve on
     the inflating bulb has been fully opened.

(3) First screening examination:

     If the mean of the two readings equals or exceeds 200 systolic or
     90 diastolic, recall one week later for second screening; otherwise
     reassure and dismiss.

(4) Second screening examination:

     The second screening examination should preferably be carried out
     1 week after the first, and not later than 4 weeks after the first.
     Take 2 further readings.
     If the mean of the 4 readings (2 at first and 2 at second screening
     examination) is less than 200 systolic and 90 diastolic reassure
     and dismiss.

     If the mean equals or exceeds 200 systolic and 110 diastolic do NOT
     enter into trial but refer for treatment.

Entry Criteria

If the mean of the 4 screening readings equals or exceeds 90 diastolic but
does not exceed 109, provided the systolic does not equal or exceed 200,
the subject should be given an appointment to see the doctor, who will
again check the blood pressure, record it on the yellow card and if suitable
will give an explanation of the trial and arrange for an entry examination
which includes ECG, blood and urine tests and a chest X-ray (optional).   If
the doctor does not confirm the BP as within the trial range, the patient
should be recalled for another set of doctor's readings.   Only if the mean
of these 4 measurements is within the range, should the patient be entered.

Record Keeping   TRIAL PROCEDURES

Records are printed in the form of a booklet for all patients referred
for the entry examination.   Each booklet is comprised of a cover (with
patient's name and trial number) and a set of forms and carbon copies,
and will provide a sequential record of all examinations made during the
first 30 months of the trial.   A supplement will be available for
patients continuing in the trial for any subsequent period of follow up.
Together, the booklet and supplement will cover the 5 year duration of
the trial.

2

The top copy of each form is retained in the booklet; carbon copies are perforated and will be detached and sent to the co-ordinating centre. For legibility, please use a black ball-point pen, make certain always to write on the top copy, and see that the carbon paper is correctly positioned.

On pages FIVE AND SEVEN you will note that there is a space allowed for the data in connection with 3 separate examinations on 3 separate occasions. Each of these pages is followed by 3 perforated sheets for carbon copies. After each examination please detach the carbon copy showing the data for the current examination, and post to the co-ordinating centre.

To avoid repeated memoranda, please check each copy for legibility and completeness; it is easier to do this while the patient is still beside you and can provide the missing information.

Notes on the completion of record forms

General Comment: Each question should receive an answer which will either be an abbreviation (Yes = Y; No = N; etc.) or a numerical digit, and each box is numbered for card punching. If the required information cannot be provided, please write NA (not available) beside the appropriate box.

Each box should contain ONE letter or ONE digit,
e.g. trial number 1 is coded

| 0 | 0 | 1 |

   diastolic pressure 84 is coded

| 0 | 8 | 4 |

Please always 'round down', i.e. record to nearest whole number below observed measurement unless the observed measurement is an integer.

e.g. 72.8 Kg should be coded:

| 0 | 7 | 2 | (not 073)

Decimal figures are used only when a decimal point is provided between boxes.

e.g. Serum Potassium 4.6 is coded:

| 4 | . | 6 |

Where the boxes are shaded, they are reserved for use by the co-ordinating centre. Please do not code in a shaded box.

<u>PAGES ONE AND TWO</u>   <u>ENTRY EXAMINATION</u>

CARD   COL.NO.

1   1-10   Identification   The identification number is
                                    only allocated when the patient
                                    is entered into the trial.
                                    <u>DO NOT COMPLETE BOXES 1-10 UNTIL</u>
                                    <u>PATIENT HAS BEEN SHOWN TO BE</u>
                                    <u>ELIGIBLE FOR ENTRY.</u>

        11-24   Surname   Block capitals, please, starting
                                    from the left, thus:

| R | O | B | I | N | S | O | N | | | | | | |

        25   Other names –
                 up to the
        26   number of two

| T | H | O | M | A | S | | | | |

| C | L | I | V | E | | | | | |

                                    Insert full forenames (up to the
                                    number of two) as shown, but the
                                    computer will use only initial
                                    letters.

1   27-32   Date of birth   Please give complete date, and record
                                    e.g. 8/4/32 as

| 0 | 8 | 0 | 4 | 3 | 2 |

        33   Marital status   Code as indicated
                                    i.e.   S, M, W, or 0

1   33   NHS Number   Please obtain the full NHS number <u>not</u>
                                    the Social Security (National Insurance)
                                    number.   This is important: it is
                                    required for follow-up through NHS
                                    records kept at Southport.

        34   Employment   Record name of factory, shop, department,
                                    etc. to facilitate follow-up.   Code
                                    employment status as indicated,
                                    i.e. G, R, S, 0 or H.

        35-46   BP at screening   Please transfer the <u>first</u> corrected
                                    (not the first mean corrected) screening
                                    BP measurements into boxes 35-49, and
                                    the mean of the 4 screening measurements
                                    into boxes 41-46.

        47,48   Observer's code   Insert a code number (e.g. 01, 02, etc.)
                                    which each person responsible for
                                    measurements should be allocated at the
                                    clinic.
                                    Boxes 47 and 48 are not used when
                                    mobile screening vans have been involved.

4

<u>Medical History and Symptoms</u>

This section covers the previous medical history and current symptoms.
The questions are designed to provide information relevant to the trial
but can allow a general assessment of the patient's health which could be
of value for follow-up purposes. Please remember to supplement answers,
where necessary, by giving additional information in Section X at the
foot of page ONE.

CARD   COL.NO.

2	17,18	Treatment for hypertension	Consider specific antihypertensive agents only; disregard sedatives, tranquillizers and dietary treatment. Previous treatment for hypertension, provided there has been no treatment within the last 3 months, is not a ground for exclusion. Please specify dates of treatment and its nature.
	19	Angina pectoris	The diagnosis should be based on the criteria of the Rose Questionnaire (a copy of which is provided at each clinic). Pain, discomfort, pressure or heaviness in the chest occuring on exertion, which requires the individual to stop or slow down, and which is then relieved in 10 min. or less.
	20	Myocardial infarction	Accept as definite a history of acute, intense retrosternal pain of constrictive, crushing or burning character frequently radiating to neck, jaw, interscapular area, shoulders. or arms - of one or more hours duration with or without ECG or enzymatic confirmation. Do not accept an atypical history unless confirmed by ECG or enzyme changes. Confirm by contacting the GP or hospital concerned.
	21	Congestive failure or cardiac asthma	Accept as definite a history confirmed by GP or hospital - in the absence of such confirmation, do not exclude unless there are physical signs suggesting failure (see below).
	22	Other heart disorder	Code as indicated. C, R, H or O as shown in patient's record booklet.
	23	Peripheral artery disease	Code as 'Yes' if satisfying criteria of Rose questionnaire (q.v.)
	24	Transient ischaemic attack	A reversible, focal, neurological deficit of less than 24 hours duration.

CARD	COL.NO.		
2	24	Hypertensive encephalopathy	Unlikely to be encountered but typically accompanied by severe headache, confusion and epileptiform fits.
		Stroke	Accept as definite a history of hemiplegia or gross hemiparesis lasting 24 hours or more. Confirm with GP or hospital unless there are residual signs.
	25	Other CNS Symptoms	Record vision defects which are uncorrected by refraction, disturbances of balance or evidence of neurological disease.
	26	Psychiatric disorder	Use judgment concerning severity - do not enter into the trial a subject unlikely to accept regular drug therapy for hypertension.
	27	Renal disease	Do not enter a patient whose hypertension appears to be secondary to recognised renal disease.
	28	Bronchial asthma	Do not enter a patient with a typical history.
	29	Chronic bronchitis	Record if cough and phlegm present for as much as 3 months each year.
	30	Other respiratory disease	Record dyspnoea as present if subject is out of breath while walking with others of same age on the level.
	31-34	Alimentary system	Record symptoms as a baseline for possible drug side effects.
	35	Diabetes	Do not enter if subject has a confirmed history of diabetes.
	36	Gout	Do not enter if subject has a confirmed history of acute attacks of gout.
	37	Other	Record presence of any other metabolic or endocrine disorder likely to be relevant to admission to trial.
	38	Arthritis	Record any arthritic symptoms which might have relevance to side effects.
	39	Other	Record any other relevant abnormality of musculo-skeletal system.

CARD   COL.NO.

| 2 | 40 | Drug allergy | Record any history of drug allergy or toxicity. |

Any Other Relevant symptoms?   Record any further information which you consider would be useful for follow-up purposes.

41   For females only   This question concerning the contraceptive pill is asked in order to allow investigation of its relationship with cardiovascular complications.   Hypertensive women on the pill should be encouraged to change to some other method of contraception; only if they are unwilling to cease using the pill, or if their BP remains high after changing to some other form of contraception, should they enter the trial. Any such change of management should be done in consultation with the GP.

42-44   Smoking   Information is required on current cigarette smoking only.   A person smoking less than 1 cigarette/day is considered a non-smoker.

Physical Examination

| 3 | 1-8 | Identification number | Reinsert name.   DO NOT INSERT NUMBER YET. |

11-17   Body weight   Record weight in Kg. (if scale is so graduated) in boxes 11-13 or in stones and lbs (if scale is so graduated) in 14-17.   Measure in light clothing (i.e. remove jackets and shoes.)

18-23   Height   Record height (no shoes) in cm (if scale is so graduated) in boxes 18-20, or in ft. and ins. (if scale is so graduated) in boxes 21-23.

24   Cardiac rhythm   Check regularity of pulse, and code as indicated.

25   Murmurs or abnormal heart sounds   Check for evidence of valvular heart disease or gallop rhythm.   Auscultate also for râles and rhonchi.

26   Cardiac failure   Consider present if patient gives a history of paroxysmal nocturnal dyspnoea, dyspnoea at rest or orthopnoea and any two of the following signs are present - râles, ankle oedema, hepatomegaly, pleural effusion, raised venous pressure, gallop rhythm, tachycardia 120 beats/ minute or more.

7

CARD	COL.NO.		
3	27	CNS signs	Examine for neurological defects - aphasia or dysarthria, tongue deviation, facial asymmetry, abnormal gait, abnormal reflexes, etc. Specify findings if any.

28   Fundi   Use Keith-Wagener classification, and code
                               findings in most affected eye, as indicated.

                               Grade I = retinal vessels with mild
                               narrowing or sclerosis.

                               Grade II = retinal vessels with moderate
                               or marked sclerosis with arterio-venous
                               nipping.

                               Grade III or IV = with cotton wool exudates,
                               haemorrhages or papilloedema. DO NOT ENTER
                               A PATIENT WITH GRADE III OR IV FUNDI. If
                               possible get a funduscopic examination
                               confirmed by second physician before excluding.

29   Other symptoms -   Record if present.
        bronchospasm   Specify any other significant abnormal findings.

33-54   Pulse and blood   One pulse count is sufficient. If a yellow
        pressure   card with the doctor's BP measurements has
        readings   been completed, please transfer the measurements.
                               If not, the doctor should measure BP twice, and
                               record readings under 1 and 2. If the
                               physician's examination gives a blood pressure
                               mean above or below the specified levels,
                               random allocation should be postponed until
                               the results of a second examination by the
                               physician are available. If the mean of these
                               4 measurements is above 110 or below 90 do not
                               enter into trial.

55-56   Observer Code   Physician's code to be entered here. Take a
        ECG   12-lead recording in a comfortable room
                               temperature, preferably (but not essentially)
                               2 or more hours after a meal, using standard
                               2.5 cm/sec paper speed. Record at least 3
                               technically good complexes for each lead, and
                               a longer strip if an arrhythmia is present.
                               Always include a 1 mv calibration signal on each
                               patient's tracing, label the leads, and write
                               the patient's name(s) and identification number,
                               and the date on each tracing. Tracings should
                               be either mounted on card (3 complexes per lead),
                               folded (uncut) into a labelled envelope, (ECG and
                               envelope can be labelled with tear-off labels
                               supplied) or, preferably, cut into 4 strips (as
                               shown in illustration on page 9) and inserted
                               into transparent plastic display covers. These
                               covers should be re-used after they have been
                               returned by the co-ordinating centre.

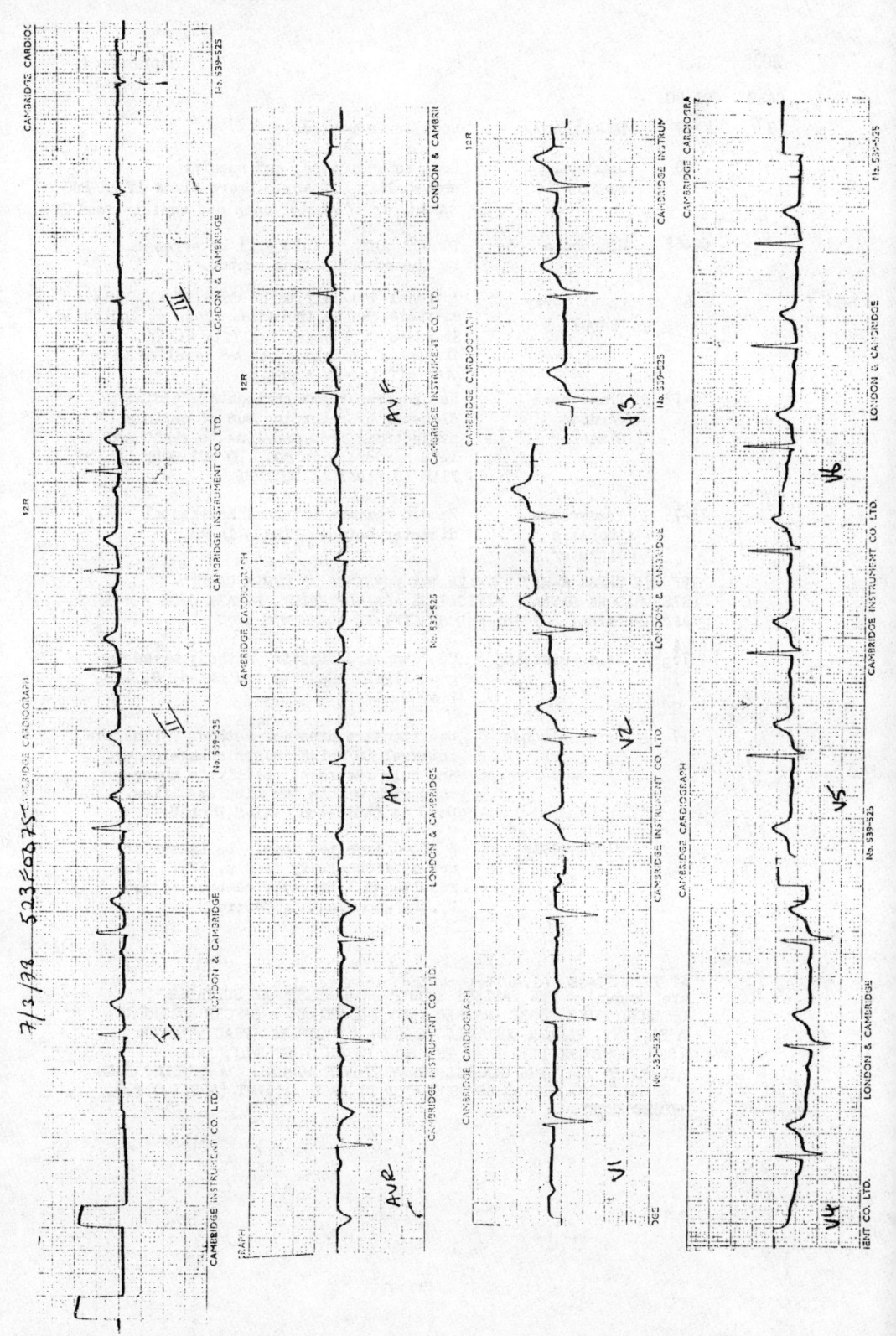

CARD	COL.NO.		
3	57	ECG taken?	Code as indicated.
	58	Clinical reading	Code as indicated, and specify abnormality, if any. Leave blank if no ECG taken, or if doctor does not want to read ECG.
	59-68	Minnesota code	DO NOT CODE. - This will be arranged by the co-ordinating centre.
	69	Chest X-ray taken?	Optional and only to be done if all trial entrants can be included. Code as indicated. Standard full sized P-A film at 6ft. tube distance. Envelope can be labelled with tear-off labels supplied.
	70-72	Transverse cardiac diameter	Record transverse horizontal cardiac diameter by recording sum of maximum projections from mid-line to right and left borders - in mm. DO NOT CODE IF FILM IS MARKEDLY ROTATED.
	73-75	Transverse thoracic diameter	Record maximum internal horizontal diameter between ribs - in mm.

IF THE CHEST X-RAY REVEALS THE PRESENCE OF OTHER CARDIO-RESPIRATORY DISEASE MITIGATING AGAINST ENTRY, PLEASE CODE APPROPRIATELY BOX 78, AND SPECIFY IN 'COMMENTS'.

	76	Urine protein	Use standard dipstick method; read in good light. Code as indicated, N, T, P or U.
	77	Urine glucose	Use standard dipstick method. Time the interval in which colour change occurs and only record as positive a change occurring within the time specified. Code as indicated, N,L,M,D or U.
		Blood tests	A blood specimen should be taken for serum biochemistry (see p. 12). The results will be reported back to you by the Coordinating Centre.

AT THIS STAGE (i.e. before the blood results are known) THE PATIENT SHOULD BE ASSESSED AS SUITABLE OR UNSUITABLE TO BE ENTERED INTO THE TRIAL.   BEFORE ENTERING A PATIENT, PLEASE COMMUNICATE WITH HIS GENERAL PRACTITIONER (SEE SUGGESTED LETTER AT THE BACK OF THIS MANUAL), AND ASCERTAIN THAT THE GENERAL PRACTITIONER AGREES.   A CONSENT FORM (SEE PAGE 20) SHOULD BE COMPLETED BY EACH PATIENT (& HIS G.P.) BEFORE ENTRY.

ALLOCATION OF TREATMENT

This will be carried out according to lists of numbers which will be prepared by the co-ordinating centre and pre-circulated to each participating clinic. Separate lists of numbers will be produced for each age/sex group and each clinic. Each list will be comprised of serial numbers; against each number will be a check letter, a code representing the basic drug regime which will be allocated to the patient, and space to enter the patient's name.

New lists of numbers will be sent to each clinic before the old ones are fully used. Further supplies of tablets for subjects not yet entered will be sent to each clinic as new lists of numbers are provided. Further supplies of tablets will also be sent automatically before a patient should be running short. The co-ordinating centre will not be providing labelled containers of supplementary drugs.

When a person is judged suitable for entry, please code box number 78, and enter his or her name opposite the next available number on the list for that person's age/sex group. Record the number and check letter in boxes 1 - 8 on PAGE ONE and at the head of PAGE TWO.

Record in boxes 4, 11-21 (foot of PAGE TWO) date of entry, treatment regime code, and the number of tablets dispensed. Insert date of next appointment.

Identification numbers

The identification number will consist of a 7 figure number plus a check letter. On all punch cards, the number will be arranged as follows:-

Cols. 1 - 2   Centre (clinic) number. Serial numbers will be allocated to each participating clinic (01,02 etc.). All reports originating from one clinic should carry this number.

3   Age-group at entry - refers to the age group to which the patient belongs on the date of entry - code as indicated, i.e. 1,2,3 or 4.

4   Sex - M for males, F for females.

5 - 7   Trial number. A 3 digit serial number (the next available number on the list mentioned under 'Allocation of treatment') - 001, 002 etc.

8   Check letter. Each number is further identified by a check letter which must be considered as part of the identification number and always entered in the records as such.

A patient's number will therefore consist of 3 digits, a letter, 3 more digits and another letter: (for example, the number 083M015H would be in clinic 08, 45-54 (the third age group), male and the fifteenth to be entered in that group. H is the check letter).

Blood Tests

Having entered the patient to the trial a 15 ml blood specimen should be
taken and transferred into a centrifuge tube; a supply of centrifuge
tubes will be sent to each participating clinic. Specimens should be
centrifuged at 2000 rpm or more between 30 mins. and 1½ hours of collection
and the serum transferred to a serum tube using Pasteur pipettes provided.
If red cells are inadvertently transferred at this stage - repeat
centrifugation. The serum tube should be labelled with name, trial number
and date. Unless serum specimens are fully identified with patient's
name and trial number the source of the specimen cannot easily be ascertained
and this therefore slows down the reporting of results.

The serum specimen is despatched to Wolfson Research Laboratories, Birmingham,
in the polystyrene pack[+]provided by the coordinating centre, using the
Business Reply Service. The coloured punch card must be included in each
pack, and is used by the Wolfson Laboratories for identification. Please
complete the patient's number (exactly as illustrated below) and name on
the card whenever a specimen is sent to Birmingham. There is no need to
complete both sides of the card.

QUEEN ELIZABETH MEDICAL CENTRE - WOLFSON LABORATORIES

REGISTRATION / CLINIC NO.
3 F 0 0 1 E

SEX   PROJECT NO
F   M 0 7

SURNAME
J O N E S

FORENAMES   AGE YRS
J A   4 7

Q.E. USE ONLY - LABORATORY NUMBER

IBM C8R- 28512

PLEASE
COMPLETE
BOTH
SIDES
OF CARD

DATE OF
COLLECTION: 14.3.77   TIME OF
                           COLLECTION :

SPECIAL PROJECT REQUEST

		TICK BELOW
1	BIOCHEMICAL PROFILE	[ ]
2	FASTING LIPID PROFILE	[ ]
3	CHOLESTEROL AND TRIGLYCERIDE (NON-FASTING SPECIMEN)	[ ]
	HAEMATOLOGY PROFILE	[ ]
5	OTHER TESTS (SPECIFY BELOW)	[ ]

QUEEN ELIZABETH HOSPITAL

* For Wolfson Laboratories purposes, the trial project code is M followed
by the clinic number; for the purpose of identification by the clinic,
the patient's number in this case is 073F001E.

Specimens should be posted by 1st class letter post the same day. Only in
exceptional circumstances should specimens be stored overnight but if this
is necessary, please store in a refrigerator at 4°C.

The results of blood tests will be transmitted to each clinic by the
coordinating centre. In the event of a blood test result disqualifying
a patient from the trial, this fact will be communicated to the clinic
by the coordinating centre.

[+] The polystyrene boxes can accommodate two serum tubes. When possible please
despatch 2 specimens (and therefore 2 cards) together, thereby saving postage.

Grounds for Exclusion

(1) Hypertension due to known underlying cause.

(2) Treatment for hypertension within the preceding 3 months.

(3) If normally accepted indications for therapy are present, eg. GRADE III or IV fundal changes, renal or cardiac failure.

(4) Confirmed myocardial infarction or cerebrovascular accident within previous three months. ECG evidence of silent myocardial infarction or left bundle branch block.

(5) Current symptoms of angina or intermittent claudication.

(6) Other serious diseases - eg. malignancy, cirrhosis, severe neurological disorder.

(7) Presence of pregnancy, diabetes, gout, asthma or heart block.

(8) Psychiatric disease.

(9) Blood potassium of 3.4 mg/100 ml or less; blood urea of 8.3 m mol (50mg/100 ml) or more.

(10) Refusal or inability of subject to attend regularly, or unwillingness of patient's G.P. to sanction therapy in the trial.

Dispensing of tablets

Bulk issues of tablets, in labelled containers of 100 each, will be issued to each clinic from the coordinating centre. There are four basic regimes - diuretic, β-blocker, two placebos similar in appearance and taste to their active counterparts.

The four tablet regimes will be numbered, and the numbering systems will be made known to those in charge of the clinics. A batch number will be printed on each label. The last digit indicates the drug regime of the tablets in the container.

Drug schedules

The primary drug regimes are as follows:

Bendrofluazide (5 mg. tablets). Basic dose 5 mg b.d.

Placebo for bendrofluazide (similar tablets). Dose 1 tablet b.d.

Propranolol (40 mg bisected tablets). Start with test dose of 20 mg, if no side effects occur increase to 20 mg b.d. for two weeks, then increase if necessary to 40 mg b.d. for 2 weeks, then if necessary to 80 mg b.d. for two weeks and then to 120 mg b.d. The dose can be increased further but only, please, after discussion with the coordinating centre. (80 mg tablets will be provided when necessary).

Placebo for propranolol (similar tablets) - basic dose and initiation of tablets as for propranolol.

Each subject, on entry, will have tablets dispensed in containers of 100; the containers will be labelled with the patient's number.

13

The aim of therapy is to control the diastolic pressure below 90 mm Hg. A patient showing a response at 12 weeks (i.e. pressure lower than at entry but not below 95 mm) can be continued on the primary drug, but should be followed up monthly with the possibility then of adding a supplementary drug. If the pressure is showing a very limited, or no response, by 8 weeks, please consider introducing the supplementary drug at that stage. It is the job of the clinic to keep an intelligent eye on dose adjustment and introduction of supplementary drugs.

Supplementary drugs

For both bendrofluazide and propranolol the first choice of supplementary drug is methyl dopa initially at a dose of 250 mg.

IT IS TO THE ADVANTAGE OF THE TRIAL TO TRY TO KEEP THE GROUPS INITIALLY ON BENDROFLUAZIDE OR ON PROPRANOLOL AS DISTINCT AND AS LARGE AS POSSIBLE, i.e. WITH AS LITTLE CONTAMINATION BY PEOPLE WHO HAVE TAKEN BOTH THESE DRUGS AS IS FEASIBLE.

If the combination of the randomly allocated primary drug and methyl dopa does not achieve good control, patients can be given supplementary guanthedine (initially at a dose of 10 mg mane). The titration of doses of these supplementary drugs is left to the clinician in charge.

Supplies of methyl dopa and guanethidine are provided for use as supplements. When needed, these should be labelled with the individual's name, number, etc. at the clinic.

Further supplies of tablets will be despatched automatically by the co-ordinating centre both for patients already in the trial and for future recruits to the trial.

BULK ISSUES OF TABLETS SHOULD BE CLEARLY IDENTIFIED AND STORED UNDER LOCK AND KEY. LABELS ON EACH CONTAINER SHOULD NOT BE REMOVED.

Having completed the ENTRY EXAMINATION, please despatch carbon copies of PAGES ONE and TWO to the co-ordinating centre.

Follow-up Examinations

Routine follow-up examinations are at fortnightly intervals for 12 weeks* then at 3-monthly intervals for the remainder of the first year, and thereafter at 6-monthly intervals. Facilities should be made to allow intervening visits, especially during the run-in period when changes in treatment may be needed, or when the pressure is inadequately controlled. Some clinics find extra visits between the 6-monthly intervals are helpful in reducing lapse rates. Proformata for 'extra visits' are provided in the form of pads. Please send data after each such visit - i.e. do not wait to complete the form.

*These fortnightly follow-up visits are not all obligatory, but should be included if possible. If some visits are to be omitted, these should be the 2-week follow-up (for those on thiazides but not for those on propranolol) and the 6, 8 and 10-week follow-up visits.

For analytical purposes, the visits at 4 weeks and 12 weeks are considered essential and should not be omitted.

Once entry dates are received at the coordinating centre a computerised list of follow-up dates and procedures will be sent for each patient's record booklet.

<u>PAGE THREE</u>

To be used for the first three fortnightly (2, 4 and 6 weeks) follow-up examinations.

Cards 5, 6 or 7   Cols. 1-8   Insert identification number.
                    11-16   Insert date of examination.
                    17   Code if there has been any change in therapy during the interval since last visit.
                    18-20   Enter number of tablets dispensed last visit.
                    21-23   Enter number of tablets remaining.
                    24-26   The difference of these two measurements gives the number taken.

A note should be made concerning the patient's compliance with the regime prescribed.

                    27   <u>Symptoms</u>   This section is to be used for symptoms volunteered. If necessary, probe for possible side effects and code as indicated, in column 28.
                           <u>Comments</u>   Please include any comment which may facilitate follow-up.
                    29   Code 'yes' if concurrent medication is being taken regularly and specify its nature.
                    30-32   Code number of days off work sick, since last appointment.
                    33-54   Record pulse, and two sets of BP measurements and note down zero errors. For clinic purposes, write in true (i.e. corrected) systolic and diastolic pressures and calculate the means of the two readings of systolic and diastolic pressure.
                    55,56   Insert observer's code.
                    57-62   Write in date of next appointment,
                    63   treatment regime prescribed (including dosage details on the dotted lines), and
                    64   whether supplementary drug is required. Again, insert the number of tablets dispensed (which may be the same as the number of tablets remaining - coded in 21-23 above).

When the 6 week examination is completed, detach carbon copy and send it to the coordinating centre.

<u>PAGE FOUR</u>

To be used for the remaining three fortnightly (8, 10 and 12 weeks) follow-up visits.

Cards 8, 9, 10   Complete and code as for PAGE THREE, but remember to repeat blood test for serum electrolytes (Na and K) only for those on diuretics, at the 12 week examination.

                                 When the 12 week examination is completed, detach carbon copy and send it to the coordinating centre.

15

Side effects questionnaire
_____

A self-administered questionnaire on side effects should be handed out
(N.B. different versions for the two sexes) and completed by the patient
at the 12 week examination.   Please check that it has been properly
filled in and despatch it with PAGE 4.

PAGE FIVE

Cards 11, 12, 13   To be used for the three quarterly
examinations (at 6, 9 and 12 months).

Complete and code as for PAGES THREE AND
FOUR but detach carbon copy after each
examination and send to coordinating centre.

Blood pressure measurements at the 12 month
visit should be recorded by the observer who
carries out routine follow-up clinics rather
than by the physician who is carrying out the
annual follow-up examination (unless, of
course, these are the same person).

AFTER DETACHING CARBON COPY PLEASE REMEMBER
TO RE-ENTER IDENTIFICATION NUMBER AT HEAD
OF SUCCEEDING COLUMN.

PAGE SIX   -   FIRST 'ANNUAL' EXAMINATION

The 'Annual' examinations are similar to, but somewhat shorter than the
entry examinations and require a similar set of routine investigations.
The carbon copy of the first annual examination should be returned to the
coordinating centre with an ECG.   If the patient is not judged suitable
to continue in the trial, a 'Withdrawal from randomised therapy' form
should also be returned.

In completing this first annual examination form, please give details of
the medical history WITHIN the last year only.

A blood sample should be taken, centrifuged, and despatched to the
Wolfson Research Laboratories, Edgbaston, Birmingham, using the Business
Reply Service.   Please remember to complete the coloured punch card.

The results will be returned to the clinic via the coordinating centre.

Repeat biochemical tests
_____

For those on bendrofluazide, the development of a Serum K level of 2.4
or 2.5 is an indication for monthly serum electrolyte determinations.
until it rises again to 2.6 or above.

The development of a Serum K level of 2.3 or below (if confirmed) is an
indication for withdrawal from randomised treatment.

16

PAGE SEVEN

To be used for the three six-monthly examinations at 18, 24 and 30 months.
Complete and code as for PAGE FIVE, and detach carbon copy after each
examination and send to coordinating centre.

AFTER DETACHING CARBON COPY, PLEASE REMEMBER TO RE-ENTER IDENTIFICATION
NUMBER AT HEAD OF SUCCEEDING COLUMN.

At 24 months, complete SECOND ANNUAL EXAMINATION (PAGE EIGHT).   This is
a similar form to that used for the FIRST ANNUAL EXAMINATION (PAGE SIX).

Supplementary booklets for follow-up examinations from 36-60 months will
be sent automatically when needed.

TERMINATION OF A PATIENT'S PARTICIPATION IN THE TRIAL

The only reasons for this are:-

(1)   Death   )
(2)   Myocardial infarction   )   Complete form notifying a terminating
(3)   Cerebrovascular accident)   event and despatch to coordinating centre.

WITHDRAWAL FROM RANDOMISED TREATMENT

Randomised therapy is discontinued for:-

(1) Those developing diastolic pressure (mean of two measurements) of
     115 mm Hg or more if confirmed at additional recall visit two weeks
     later.

(2) Those developing systolic pressure of 210 mm Hg or more (mean of two
     measurements) if confirmed at additional recall visit 2 weeks later.

(3) Those developing mean pressures of these levels on 3 or more
     occasions (but not necessarily consecutive).

     Patients in the above categories who were previously receiving
     placebo tablets should be transferred to the corresponding
     active drug.

(4) Development of renal failure, cardiac failure, hypertensive retinopathy
     or encephalopathy. Discontinue randomised treatment, notify
     coordinating centre and arrange appropriate therapy for each individual.

(5) Development of angina if it cannot be adequately controlled without
     antihypertensive drugs.

(6) Development of ECG evidence of infarction (submit ECG to coordinating
     centre).

(7) Development of adverse side effects (evidence to be sent or telephoned
     to coordinating centre before withdrawal from randomised therapy).

(8) Discontinuation of taking tablets, defaulting, leaving area (to a part
     of the country where there is no trial clinic) or leaving factory
     employment.

Under all these circumstances, please complete a form notifying withdrawal from randomised therapy and despatch to coordinating centre.   Keep copy in patient's record book.

All subjects who have once entered the trial, including those withdrawn from randomised therapy and those suffering a non-fatal terminating event, should be followed-up in the usual trial way, if at all possible.   If patient is known to have suffered a terminating event (death, myocardial infarction, or cerebrovascular accident) following withdrawal from randomised treatment, a form notifying the terminating event should also be completed and sent to the coordinating centre.

Soliciting consent from general practitioners and participants

It is suggested that industrial clinics should use a letter, along the lines set out on page 19, which should be sent to each potential participant's general practitioner before entering a patient into the trial.   It is essential that each patient should be given a brief explanation of the nature of the trial and be asked to sign a consent form, a version of which is shown on page 20.

Sickness absence

A period of sickness absence from normal duties of 21 days or more should be notified to the coordinating centre.   'No carbon required' (NCR) forms for doing this will be circulated to each clinic.   These are shown on page 21.   The top sheet of these forms should be sent to the coordinating centre and the copy inserted in the patient's record booklet.

Notification of withdrawal from randomised treatment and Notification of a terminating event

The forms for these are also on NCR paper and are shown on pages 22 and 23. Again, top sheets, please, to the coordinating centre, copies to the patient's notes.

When information has to be solicited from hospitals this can generally be done by the coordinating centre, and a copy of the letter which will be used for this purpose is shown on page 24.

Notification of family physician of nature of therapy

It is important to inform the patient's GP of the nature of the therapy prescribed in the trial, and to remind him to keep this information from the patient.

Trial identification cards

A trial identification card which fits into a small transparent plastic wallet should be given to each patient who enters the trial. Copies of each side of the card are shown on page 25.

Requisitioning of further supplies of tablets, serum packs, etc.

Forms for requesting re-supplies are available and should be completed and despatched to the coordinating centre monthly (or quarterly).   Please allow at least two weeks for preparation and delivery.

18

Dear Dr.

We have been asked by the Medical Research Council to collaborate in a multicentre treatment trial for mild hypertension and have been screening our employees with a view to detecting untreated hypertension

One of your patients ....

of   ....

....

has been found - after three sets of screening measurements - to have a persistently raised pressure, and though this is not at a level where therapy is definitely indicated, your patient is considered eligible to be entered into a controlled trial.

The trial is designed to determine whether prolonged treatment (5 years) for those with diastolic pressures within the range 90 - 109 Hg reduces morbidity and mortality.   Patients who are entered into the trial are told that they have an equal chance of being treated with act or inert tablets, but all will be regularly examined and anyone found subsequently to need it will be given active therapy.

We do not wish to increase your work load and would suggest, if y are agreeable, that we might take over the responsibility for further investigation, treatment and follow up of your patient's hypertension. We would, of course, refer to you any condition we might find other tha hypertension.

You may feel there are specific circumstances which would render your patient's admission to the trial undesirable.   If you do feel thi would be most grateful if you would let me know, by letter or telephone call, at the above address.   If we do not hear from you we shall assum that you have no objection to your patient being included in the trial will proceed to initiate treatment.   We will keep you informed of the details of treatment and would ask you <u>not</u> to divulge these to your pat unless there is an over-riding reason for doing so.

                                   Yours sincerely,

PATIENT'S SURNAME (please print) ....

PATIENT'S TRIAL NUMBER ....

MRC TREATMENT TRIAL FOR MILD HYPERTENSION
CONSENT FORM

It is possible that treatment might help people whose blood pressure is
only mildly elevated above normal values.

We are helping the Medical Research Council to conduct a trial to assess
the need for treatment in such cases and your blood pressure has been
found to be at a level where tablets might benefit you.

All who are enrolled into the trial will be kept under regular medical
supervision and will receive either one of several different kinds of
tablet, some of which have no effect, or careful observation only.
Anyone whose blood pressure is found to rise to levels where there is no
doubt that treatment is beneficial would be withdrawn from the trial and
given appropriate treatment.

We would be grateful if you would sign the accompanying form if you are
willing to enter the trial.   Obviously, you can withdraw at any stage if
you wish.

I have read the above explanation and the nature of the trial has been

explained orally to me and I have had an opportunity of asking any

questions.   It is on the basis of the explanation and the information in

this form that I agree to participate in the blood pressure treatment

trial.

                    Signed ....

                    Date   ....

Family physician's agreement

I am the general practitioner of the above patient and in my opinion there

is nothing in the medical history to contraindicate entry into the trial.

The patient would enter the trial with my consent.

                    Signed ....

                    Date   ....

NO CARBON
REQUIRED

MRC TREATMENT TRIAL FOR MILD HYPERTENSION

NOTIFICATION OF SICKNESS ABSENCE OF 21 DAYS OR LONGER

It is essential that these forms be completed for all trial participants on return to work, or on leaving employment after an illness of 21 days or more.

NAME ....

TRIAL NUMBER   ⬚⬚⬚⬚⬚⬚ ⬚

Date of first day of absence ....

Date of return to work/leaving employment ....

Diagnosis (as written on certificate) ....

Name of general practitioner ....

             (Inpatient
Attended hospital (Outpatient   (Please underline whichever applies)
             (Neither

If hospital attended: Name of hospital ....

                   Name of consultant ....

Other relevant information ....

....

....

....

....

....

PLEASE DETACH TOP COPY AND POST TO:-

    MRC/DHSS EPIDEMIOLOGY AND MEDICAL CARE UNIT, NORTHWICK PARK HOSPITAL,
          WATFORD ROAD, HARROW, MIDDLESEX HA1 3UJ

NO CARBON
REQUIRED   MRC TREATMENT TRIAL FOR MILD HYPERTENSION

                NOTIFICATION OF WITHDRAWAL FROM RANDOMISED TREATMENT

NAME .... NUMBER [| | | | | |] [ ]   1- 8

CARD No.   [5][0]   9-10

DATE OF NOTIFICATION OF WITHDRAWAL FROM   [| | | | |]   11-16
    RANDOMISED TREATMENT   Day Month Year

This patient has been withdrawn from randomised
    treatment for the following reason :-

Inadequate blood pressure control   Y or N [ ]   17

Development of renal failure, cardiac failure,
    hypertensive retinopathy or encephalopathy   Y or N [ ]   18

    If 'Yes', specify ....

Onset of angina pectoris   Y or N [ ]   19

    If 'Yes', please repeat ECG and send photocopy
        to co-ordinating centre

ECG evidence of silent myocardial infarct   Y or N [ ]   20

    If 'Yes', please send photocopy to co-ordinating centre

Persistent side effects (Please do not withdraw from
    randomised treatment without previously notifying·
    co-ordinating centre)   Y or N [ ]   21

    If 'Yes', specify ....

Development of other disease militating against
    treatment   Y or N [ ]   22

Persistent failure to take prescribed tablets   Y or N [ ]   23

Other reason not noted above   Y or N [ ]   24

    If 'Yes' specify ....

Left the district and cannot be followed up   Y or N [ ]   25

    If 'Yes', please supply new address, if known

    ....

    ....

                    Signed ....

PLEASE DETACH TOP COPY AND POST IT TO CO-ORDINATING CENTRE:-
MRC/DHSS EPIDEMIOLOGY AND MEDICAL CARE UNIT, NORTHWICK PARK HOSPITAL,
            WATFORD ROAD, HARROW, MIDDLESEX HA1 3UJ

NO CARBON REQUIRED

MRC TREATMENT TRIAL FOR MILD HYPERTENSION

NOTIFICATION OF TERMINATING EVENT

NAME .... NUMBER [ ][ ][ ][ ][ ][ ][ ]   1- 8

CARD No.   [6][0]   9-10

DATE OF NOTIFICATION OF TERMINATING EVENT   [| |]   11-16
                                                Day Month Year

This patient has been withdrawn from the trial due to:-

<u>NON-FATAL MYOCARDIAL INFARCTION</u>   Y or N [ ]   17

   If 'Yes', date of infarction   [| |]   18-23
                                               Day Month Year

   Was patient admitted to hospital?   Y or N [ ]   24

      If 'Yes', which hospital? ....

      Under which consultant? ....

      If 'No', please give name and address of practitioner from whom
        further details could be obtained

      ....

      ....

<u>NON-FATAL CEREBROVASCULAR ACCIDENT</u>   Y or N [ ]   37

   If 'Yes', date of CVA   [| |]   38-43
                                               Day Month Year

   Was patient admitted to hospital?   Y or N [ ]   44

      If 'Yes', which hospital? ....

      Under which consultant? ....

      If 'No', please give name and address of practitioner from whom
        further details could be obtained

      ....

      ....

<u>DEATH</u>   Y or N [ ]   57

   If 'Yes', date of death   [| |]   58 63
                                               Day Month Year

Place of death ....

Was death sudden (i.e. within 24 hrs of onset of symptoms)?   Y or N [ ]   64

Please give certified cause of death

     Ia ....

      b ....

      c ....

     II ....

Was an autopsy performed?   Y or N [ ]   65

              Signed ....

**PLEASE DETACH TOP COPY AND POST TO MRC/DHSS EPIDEMIOLOGY AND MEDICAL CARE UNIT,
NORTHWICK PARK HOSPITAL, WATFORD ROAD, HARROW, MIDDLESEX HA1 3UJ**

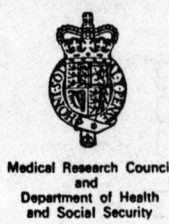

Medical Research Council
and
Department of Health
and Social Security

Epidemiology and Medical Care Unit
Northwick Park Hospital
Watford Road, Harrow
Middlesex HA1 3UJ

telephone 01-864 5311

reference

Dear Sir,

The Medical Research Council's treatment trial for mild hypertension is designed to determine whether treatment of hypertension at an early stage reduces the incidence of cardiovascular complications.

The trial is a multicentre one, in which industries, population screening programmes and general practitioners are collaborating. This Unit is acting as the co-ordinating centre.

An important feature is the monitoring of morbidity and mortality and for this reason we would be very grateful if you would send us a copy of the discharge summary of the following patient in the trial who, we understand, was recently treated at your hospital. A stamped addressed envelope is enclosed.

Name ....

Address ....

....

....

Date of birth ....

This information will remain strictly confidential.

Yours sincerely,

Specimen Trial Identification Card (with wallet)

Medical Research Council
Hypertension Research Programme

Mr/Mrs/Miss

Address

Is taking part in this programme which necessitates taking either a thiazide diuretic, a β-blocker or a placebo as a long term measure. If it becomes necessary for the nature of the treatment to be revealed, please contact the address on the reverse of this card.

reverse
side of
card

Clinic

Address

Telephone

To the patient
Please show this card if you need to attend a hospital.
Whilst on this trial you should not donate blood for transfusion purposes.

FLOW CHART FOR MRC PROTOCOL –
BP CRITERIA FOR SCREENING FOR THE MRC TRIAL

1ST VISIT → Measure blood pressure TWICE → Is the mean of the two readings 200 mm or above – systolic?

- YES → Recall for 2nd visit preferably one week but not exceeding 4 weeks later
- NO → Is the mean of the two readings 90 mm or above – diastolic?
  - YES → Recall for 2nd visit preferably one week but not exceeding 4 weeks later
  - NO → Reassure and Dismiss

Is diastolic 110 mm or above?
- YES → Do not include in Trial. Recommend for further investigation and treatment
- NO → Reassure and Dismiss

2ND VISIT → Measure blood pressure TWICE → Establish the mean systolic and diastolic of all 4 readings → Is the mean of all 4 diastolic readings between 90 mm and 109 mm?
- YES → Is diastolic 110 mm or above? → YES → Do not include in Trial. Recommend for further investigation and treatment
- NO → Is mean of all 4 systolic readings 200 mm or above?
  - YES → Do not include in Trial. Recommend for further investigation and treatment
  - NO → Refer subject to the physician who will re-check the pressure and assess eligibility for entry in the Trial.

26

Index

She gave a harsh laugh.

"Coed Bedwen. Even now, is that all you can think about?"

"What else is there?" He certainly wasn't thinking about tasting her lips, teasing them into a smile. No. She was a Comyn. He mustn't forget his oath. He forced his face into an expressionless mask and faced her.

She had blotted away her tears and was standing straight, her chin up, face composed. "Our…our marriage, for a start. We should discuss it."

"What is there to say? I already know your thoughts on the matter. You want me to die or journey to the Holy Land. Believe me, I have no intention of doing either."

Matilda winced. "So you haven't forgotten that."

"I rarely forget anything. You can be sure I'll check my food and drink very carefully from now on."

"I'd never—"

"But you did." He rubbed his temples. Tried to ignore the beguiling scent of honeysuckle. "All I want is Coed Bedwen. As the king has made it clear the only way I can achieve that is through marriage to you, then marry we must."